Addiction no More !
Chronic Pain no More !

by

John Hesnan

Addiction no More! – Chronic Pain no More!

Version1.0 - June 2016

Published by John Hesnan

(c) Copyright 2016 - John Hesnan

ISBN: 978-1539024408

This book is not designed to provide psychological advice or as a substitute for professional counselling. The information comes with no warranty, expressed or implied, with regard to the subject matter covered. It is sold with the understanding that the authors are not engaged in rendering legal, accounting, medical or other professional advice. If legal advice or other professional assistance is required, the services of a competent professional should be sought. John Hesnan, individually or corporately, does not accept any responsibility for any liabilities resulting from the actions of any parties involved. No responsibility is accepted for use of this information. Use is entirely at your own risk. Information contained is for educational purposes only.

Table of Contents

Contents

FOREWORD

"Addiction no More, Chronic Pain no More" explores the MindBody creation and cure of addiction and chronic pain through knowledge, awareness and acceptance of the cause.

When I wrote this book I had completed over 30 years of continuous sobriety, in Alcoholics Anonymous (AA), having previously survived a traumatic life of chronic alcoholism.

I now know that, like chronic pain or depression, alcoholism and other addictions can be cured permanently, and that alcoholics can drink socially without returning to alcohol addiction, or alcoholism, as it is more commonly known. I have proven this.

Alcoholism and other addictions are another form of an elaborate MindBody interaction, and like chronic pain they can be cured permanently, by taking personal control over your mind and your body, by telling your mind to change the effects you created when you first linked the drink or drug to its addictive power. At the time you did this, you probably had a very compelling reason to give this power to the drug of your choice.

With alcoholism the cure lies in education, acknowledgement and acceptance of the MindBody process of addiction. Before you go back drinking again you need to acknowledge, understand and accept this fact.

As you read this book, consider what mind-altering drug is, or was, affecting your life. It may be alcohol, food, sex, money, drugs, gambling or any other form of addiction. The content of this book is applicable to all addictions. In the case of addictions like anorexia, addiction means the addictive non-use of a substance that is necessary for maintaining life.

For those who have also suffered physical, emotional or sexual abuse as a child, this new MindBody knowledge will help them to move on with their lives and to stop giving control of their life to others. It will help to reveal and heal their pain, eliminating the unconscious creation of physical and emotional diversions in their lives, now and in the future.

I'm not involved in any religious or spiritual organisation. I neither endorse nor refute any of these organisations and believe everyone has the right to follow their own beliefs.

Read this book with an open mind. The foundations of this book are based on neuro-scientific investigation at molecular level.

CHAPTER 1 A MindBody Creation

In this book I will attempt to add a new chapter to the working philosophy of Bill Wilson, the founder of Alcoholics Anonymous (AA).

The 12-Step recovery organization "Alcoholics Anonymous" was founded in 1939 by Bill and his alcoholic colleagues. I know that many lives have been saved, including my own, as a result of their experience and wisdom.

My recovery solution is as radical as Bill Wilson's. However, unlike Bill and his AA program, complete recovery for me from alcoholism, means being able to take a drink like any normal social drinker. This involves looking at your life in a completely new way and accepting that drink is not the problem, you are.

Bill Wilson believed that a spiritual experience was necessary for recovery from active alcoholism, and that permanent daily abstinence from alcohol was essential for the addict.

Bill's idea of accepting a power of "your own understanding" into your life, works very well for the person who never wants to drink again, even though they might have an urge or compulsion to drink. His program has been proven to work by thousands of alcoholics. It provides the alcoholic with the resources to stay off drink under any circumstances, one day at a time.

However I believe that for an alcoholic, taking a drink without the addictive nature clicking in, only happens when you go beyond Bill's spiritual idea, and move from accepting a power of your own understanding into your life, to finding that power within yourself, and living in that power, and accepting that you were always a pure being, just one who had lost their away.

With my new MindBody knowledge I began to realize that my true self has unlimited power, and is not powerless over alcohol or any other addictive substance.

I believe and have proven, that when you have the proper knowledge and full acceptance of the MindBody creation of your alcoholism (or other addiction), you will become aware of your powerful ability to change this addictive creation, using the power of your mind.

In Alcoholics Anonymous, the First Step suggests that an AA member accepts that "We are powerless over alcohol, that our lives had become unmanageable". With this acceptance of powerlessness, my life continued to be one of calamity and pain long after I had stopped drinking. With the new acceptance that I am 'powerful' over my addiction and physical pain I was able to permanently cure both.

With alcohol removed from my life other physical and emotional symptoms became big issues in my life, until I came to fully understand their origin and source as being MindBody created. I then discovered that I really did have power and control within myself to resolve these issues and cure my alcoholism as well.

In this book, you will learn to accept that when you have a right relationship with yourself, that you are powerful over alcohol and every other issue in your life, and that you can take a drink without the addictive craving for another one. You will take the power from your addictive drug of choice and take control back into your own hands, using the power of your mind.

Alcoholism and other addictions are created in the unconscious and affect your body and your brain. The compulsive addiction is often called a disease of consciousness which is inaccurate.

At the level of Being and consciousness, the addicts neediness, the addicts desires and cravings, the addicts personality, the addicts repressed emotions in the unconscious, the addicts need for recognition, the addicts need for approval from others, and the addicts longing for acceptance and respect, are the origins of the brains 'want' to create something to mimic these needs. So the brain uses your drug of choice as a diversion from repressed emotions and you cooperate with its plan.

As is well known and documented, the main physical symptoms of addiction are; strong desire, compulsion and craving. The body and brain crave the sensual stimulation from alcohol or other mind-altering substance or activity, to prevent the unconscious reservoir of painful emotions escaping into consciousness.

So for some people, repressed emotions manifest physically in the body through pain and for others they are manifested through addiction or depression.

The mind fears that the unconscious rage or other strong emotions will break out into consciousness, destroying our image of ourselves in front of others, so it finds a diversion, either physical or emotional, and sometimes both.

The earliest reasons for repressed rage and the other strong emotions that we carry inside could be from trauma in infancy and childhood. This could be from physical, emotional or sexual abuse, or simply from feeling left out, and it can occur in any family.

Also, later in your life, stressful events like the death of a spouse, divorce, personal injury or illness, relationship difficulties, grief, work issues, retirement, finances, business difficulties, moving house, etc., can cause anger and rage that we often unconsciously suppress.

Your personality traits are another reason for repression. For example if you have low self esteem, if you are a perfectionist, if you are a hostile or aggressive type of person, if you carry a lot of guilt or shame, if you are a people pleaser, or if you are over-dependant on others. Other reasons for anger and rage are that our basic needs are not being met.

In the case of alcoholism and drug addiction there is a mental and physical craving created without our conscious knowledge, to divert attention from and hide repressed emotions and prevent them from surfacing.

It is only when you realise and accept the truth of who you really are at the level of consciousness that you can reach the goal of social drinking again. As long as you continue to believe that you are a powerless solitary physical form without control over your own life or over your own mind, it is better that you do not drink again as you will allow the diversion to continue and you will keep your addiction alive.

Once you have acknowledged and accepted the source of your addiction, and understood the MindBody creation process and the reasons for it, you will then be able to live without any addiction in your life.

You will clearly see that the monster you created can be uncreated, that the addiction can be cured and cured permanently through the power of your mind. You will be able to live like any normal social drinker and take a drink or leave it as you please without the addictive compulsive switch turning on, because you have disabled it through your own power.

Without this MindBody education acknowledgement and acceptance, you will keep your addiction alive, even without a drink. You will continue to tell yourself that you have no control; that control is not in your hands.

However when you understand the MindBody interaction and how it activates physical or emotional pain and addictions in your life, and how you can access the source of this creation and prevent the cause, then and only then will you understand what it means to be totally free of addiction.

At the end of this book I have included a recovery program called "Over The Influence" or "OTI". It is a support group where members can reveal and heal the source of their addiction and pain and build a new fulfilling life with like-minded people.

I have also added some Mindfulness Meditation practices to use to reduce stressors in your life. Mindfulness Meditation is a powerful way to live in the present and to accept that you are in control of your life.

CHAPTER 2 Alcoholics Anonymous

The ideas and philosophy of Bill Wilson, in his book Alcoholics Anonymous (AA), has saved the lives of countless alcoholics and addicts throughout the world since he set up the Fellowship in the 1930s.

The AA philosophy combines abstinence from alcohol alongside a spiritual recovery program for living sober. 'Sober' in AA means staying away from alcohol for the rest of your life.

The AA program helps a person addicted to alcohol, to stop drinking and to live a reasonably sane and sober life without the use of alcohol.

The AA philosophy is based around a 12-Step spiritual recovery programme. The programme suggests that members stay away from one drink, one day at a time, go to AA meetings and complete the 12 recovery Steps outlined in the AA textbook "Alcoholics Anonymous", also called the Big Book of AA.

Over the years, the AA program has been adopted by many other self-help organisations, to aid recovery from other compulsive addictions, including drugs, sex, money, food, gambling and many more.

At its very basic level, the AA recovery programme suggests that the addicted person stops taking alcohol or other drug of choice one day at a time, completes a moral inventory of their active addictive life, makes a confession of their glaring personality defects, makes restitution to those who were harmed during their active addiction, attends AA meetings on a regular basis, and helps others to recover from alcoholism.

Although AA is a non-religious organisation and accepts all creeds and kinds who have a desire to stop drinking, it does encourage members to become willing to find a belief or dependence on a higher power or a "God of your own understanding". For agnostics and atheists this belief can be in the AA meeting itself.

The founder Bill Wilson, based on his own recovery from alcoholism, accepted that a complete psychic change of the person was required to recover from alcoholism.

For alcoholics and the medical profession, AA was the first ray of hope for this incurable disease (as it is often mistakenly called). AA continued to create miraculous results ever since the time of its foundation.

In AA, 'recovery' or 'sober' means never drinking alcohol again. For me recovery from alcoholism means being able to drink socially again without any addictive or compulsive desire for more drink.

The AA abstinence policy also holds true for many of the other 12 step fellowships which were spawned from AA; including Narcotics Anonymous, Gamblers Anonymous, and Debtors Anonymous.

Since the foundation of AA, it has been heretical to even consider that recovery for an alcoholic could mean a return to drinking like a normal social drinker. Alcoholics Anonymous and most medical organisations have agreed up to now that alcoholism is a fatal disease and can only be arrested one day at a time by not drinking alcohol.

However, like chronic pain, which I have also cured through the power of my mind, I know and have proven that alcoholism has a similar source and can be cured permanently in the same way.

For many alcoholics who have left AA and tried social drinking, the results have been horrendous and the person often ends up committing suicide, or if they are lucky they return again to AA. This frightening statistic has led mostly everyone to believe the saying that 'once an alcoholic always an alcoholic'.

For me, this statement is the equivalent of blindly saying 'once in pain, always in pain', which I reject totally and have proven to be wrong.

Every alcoholic who has been continuously sober in AA for 30 years or more, including myself, were afraid to think any different, less they be led back to addiction and to certain death, or worse, a prolonged life of alcoholic torture. I've no doubt that that is the reality for anyone who drinks again, if they do not have knowledge and acceptance of the MindBody cure for alcoholism that I am introducing here.

There is no doubt that without AA I would not have stopped drinking over 30 years ago. I am indebted to AA for saving my life. I was a chronic alcoholic with all the classic symptoms of continuous drinking, morning cures, hangovers, blackouts, 'geographicals', cravings, obsession with alcohol, delirium tremens, convulsions, alcoholic poisoning, work and money problems, getting beaten up, ending up in rehab units, numerous serious accidents, and numerous hospitalisations.

However I now know that I can go beyond Bill Wilson's idea that recovery from alcoholism means continuous abstinence from alcohol. I now know that total recovery from alcoholism is possible and an alcoholic can return to normal social drinking without any of the effects of active alcoholism. I know that this holds true for other addictions as well.

Like Bill Wilson's AA program, my cure requires a psychic change for the individual affected by addiction. It requires that you start looking at your addiction from a different angle. In many cases it will necessitate abstinence from alcohol for a period of time until the mind is clear enough to fully understand and accept this new concept.

The initial period of abstinence and return to physical and mental health following active alcoholism, especially chronic alcoholism, cannot be achieved if you substitute another mind altering substance for alcohol.

Only when you have achieved a reasonable amount of time off alcohol and clarity of mind and physical health returns, should you begin to look at this new information. Only when you understand what I'm saying, can you take control of your life and return to normal social drinking.

Once you understand the source and the process, you can leave any other addictions behind as well, when you have accepted your true self, and experienced the power and control that you do have, to influence your mind and body.

You will understand the source of your addiction and understand that you have the power to cure your addiction and other MindBody symptoms, permanently.

CHAPTER 3 Being Happy

Most people want to be happy in life. If you ask anyone, what their main concern in life is, most people will say 'to be happy' or 'happiness'.

How to be happy, how to stay happy or how to recover happiness, is the motive of all we do and of all we are willing to endure in its pursuit.

Whatever makes you happy you will try to adopt. This could be naturally induced, drug induced or some form of spiritually induced. Each of these will have very different outcomes in the long-term.

All of us are born reasonably happy and well-balanced from birth. Some of us have trauma during pregnancy, birth or during our childhood. Some will have experienced emotional, physical or sexual abuse. For the majority of people their passions are not excessive and their lives are not haunted by regrets or strong repressed emotions. They live normal happy balanced lives.

Others, like myself, had a different view of life from the time of my birth, what I would like to call my first birth. My life from day one ranged from days of unusual fears to ones of extreme unhappiness, tragedy, serious soul-searching and trauma. I always felt separate from my family and from life in general and I was constantly looking for approval.

My life seemed to be always missing something. I always felt I needed a fresh start, maybe a different family. I was always examining my motivations, continually looking at myself as if I had another persona. I felt something missing from my life. Yet to the outside world I was a fairly happy-go-lucky type of person, with pretty normal social skills.

From infancy, I became very good at repressing my insecurities and fears so that they were not visible to others. For many years I searched painfully in places outside of myself to try and find the missing piece of my personal jigsaw, to find what I felt was the void in my life.

After years of personal pain, through mental and physical torture from chronic alcoholism, I found my first opening, an avenue to what I now call a second birth.

And 30 years later, after continuous sobriety in AA, another revelation opened up to what I call my third birth. I realized what the haunting, separateness, guilt and low self-worth throughout my life were related to and why I kept repeating the same patterns in my life.

After many years in the throes of alcoholism and after 30 years without taking any alcohol, I truly began to understand for the first time how to take control of my own life.

I was very lucky to survive the painful journey with and without alcohol, to where I now accept life as it is. I've been very fortunate to be able to heal my physical, emotional and addictive pains and turn my life around.

If you are an addict and are lucky enough to survive the search for yourself, that is if you are like me, then with this new information you will succeed in finding a way out of your misery, your addiction, your dependence and your separateness.

I thought this would happen for me by finding a spiritual power in my life. I now know that this was just a way of not accepting responsibility for myself. It worked to keep me away from alcohol one day at a time, but by keeping me away from myself, I continued to tell myself that drinking socially was dangerous for me and I remained an addict in mind and body.

When I found my true self and found that I had control over every aspect of my life, both my mind and my physical body, I realised that I could cure my addiction completely and return to social drinking.

Until this way into life and the way out of misery is found, until this type of rebirth occurs, your mind will war with your body, wayward impulses will continually interrupt your most deliberate plans, and your life will continue to be one of major drama, of remorse, of guilt, of repentance and of continuous efforts to repair misdemeanours and mistakes in your life.

Any action or substance, whether it is alcohol, drugs, money, sex or food that is taken to find a way into what you think life is, what you think is normality, or that is taken as a rebirth substitute, that is, as a solution to a fear of some kind, becomes the problem itself rather than the solution.

In itself it creates new fears and an endless searching for some other fix to cure the fear and separateness in your life. This is the early-stage formation of addiction.

By giving the substance or action, or inaction, the energy of a solution, you give it the power to create addiction in your life because it will never become the solution you want.

You are always the problem and you are always the solution. You were the starting point for addiction, for the creation of your mental health and your physical health. You are the starting point for your new power and the starting point for freedom from addiction, for freedom from pain, and for freedom from every other dysfunctional issue in your life.

You were the starting point for everything that happened in your life. You may not have been the cause but you are the creator, the creator of your alcoholism, of your despair, of your addictions, and you are the starting point for a complete recovery and for the cure of your addiction. You have this power within you and you have to let your brain know, that you know what it has been up to.

In my early drinking life, following my initial drink-induced short-term highs, I always needed more drink to reach that same place, but drink never worked the same again, instead it let me down and created a craving for more, which is the earliest sign of addiction (called 'the phenomena of craving') by Bill Wilson in the Big Book of AA.

During my active alcoholism I addictively continued to drink more and more, in a never-ending search that led to many horrors until eventually I stopped and came into AA.

I was using alcohol, a mind-altering substance, to try to reach normality, not knowing that normality was always within me. I just did not know how to access normality or what the broken unconscious and conscious links were, that were hiding this normality from me.

When I stopped drinking, other issues, like money, had the same power of disturbance in my life. I started experiencing the same distress trying to handle these issues. I started chasing money as a solution for the void in me. And as with alcohol addiction, I give money power then chased it for a solution and the result was the same. Money was not a problem either, I was. I kept ending up in the same broken state, thinking 'How did this happen again?' This is a question every addict asks at some point in their life.

While substituting the effects of money and other addictions for the effects of drink, I was staying off alcohol. Not realising what was happening, I tried other 12 step programs. They didn't work for me. I believe this was fortunate. If they had worked, I would probably have continued to delve into other addictions, as I did not understand the source of my original addiction.

Some people who go into recovery programs often go from one Twelve Step program to another in a never-ending cycle looking for another solution to another addiction, not knowing that the solution is within them.

I have found that the solution was not in the substance, it was not in the meetings and it was not in the absence of the substance either. It was in me.

Without knowledge of the source, that is, the cause of your addiction, you will be like a planet that has spun out of control; you will smash your universe to pieces, just as I had been doing with mine all my life.

I had to learn many tough lessons during my life, but it wasn't until recent years that I came face-to-face with my repressed emotions and low self-esteem demons, as they manifested in many addiction issues.

My unconscious reservoir of repressed emotions and low self-esteem triggered a conscious neediness or craving in me to fill this unconscious lack. I used alcohol to try and fill this void and gave alcohol the power to be the void.

When addictive drinking destroyed me and was then removed from my life, other issues were substituted that had the same power and control over me, until I had the MindBody realisation that led to the cure.

Unlike the rest of my family, I was constantly looking for acceptance and approval. The early unconscious unease in me was well on the way to the unease of addiction that manifested in its physical form many years later.

As a child I always felt different. I always thought that I had been adopted. I felt apart from my family and from life in general. This was not a reflection on the love I received from my parents as I was treated the same as the rest of my siblings and none of them ended up with addiction issues. It was a reflection of my inner being.

I left home at twelve years of age to find a new life. I was constantly in fear and feeling lonely and stupid. My early fears extended into my teenage and adult life, leading to many years of loneliness, despair, chronic addiction, tragedy and trauma.

I spent most of my life searching for what I thought was missing in me, that is, the other or real self. I was always pretending to be someone I was not, and when I was myself, it was misunderstood as being cocky, so my Self was repressed, adding more painful emotions to my gradually-filling reservoir of rage.

Following years of trauma and soul-searching I discovered that I was born with what I now call a divided self. When I found what was missing and accepted it into my life, part of my life changed dramatically. Some of my addictive behaviours stopped, but others started to appear until I acknowledged and accepted the underlying MindBody origins and cause of my addictions.

Once dependence on alcohol was removed from my life, I turned my life around and became an award-winning inventor. I learned how to learn and taught others how to learn through the medium of music, using patented interactive software programs.

However it took many years of pain and trauma before I fully understood the MindBody symptoms that were manifesting and prolonging pain and addiction in my life, although I was no longer taking alcohol.

I was born after a miscarriage. It is a well-known psychological fact that the unacknowledged and unexpressed emotions of a parent following a miscarriage can be felt and carried by the next child in the womb and can become part of the next child's emotional make-up.

When a parent has not properly grieved for the last miscarried baby, they often become emotionally unavailable to fully bond with the new child, so the all-important sense of parental bonding may not happen for some children in a family. This might have led to my feeling of not been wanted or of being adopted. It really does not matter. The addiction was in me and it was up to me to find its source and to cure it.

My early-stage emotional neediness led me to continually try to prove myself, first to my parents and then carrying that same inferior unwanted feeling throughout much of my life.

This was the start of me building my unconscious reservoir of strong emotions like anger, fear, loss and abandonment. This reservoir of repressed emotions increased the feeling that I was missing something, that there was a void in my life.

This was the split, the divided self I entered the world with. I did not unify my life until I had destroyed it with addiction and then stumbled on to who I was and what I was looking for.

This may have been the origin, the psychological source of my addiction, the when and why it happened. I had been disconnected and un-bonded from my soul mates, my parents since birth and probably before birth. For other people, their addictive personality may have a completely different cause, but the traumatic effect is the same.

I believe that in my case, the reservoir of rage started to fill up before I entered the world and I carried these repressed emotions into life with me.

At birth, I was a divided human being, not full of wonder and joy, but full of concern and very aware of my surroundings.

For the first half of my life, my wellbeing was seriously affected without me understanding what was going or where it came from. From an early age I started to use the mind-altering substance, alcohol, to try and recreate something that I sensed was there before the repression started. Legal and illegal drugs are used by many for the same purpose.

So my life was a balancing act for many years between the mind and the body, unconscious, conscious and subconscious. I tried to use the natural world to regain my wellbeing and while using alcohol, pushed my life to its limits until it broke and came close to total annihilation.

For me, it was only when my natural life was destroyed that I was ready to surrender and become willing to believe there was something else going on, that there was another self that was my true bond to the happiness that eluded me all my life.

Before surrendering or accepting defeat, I waited unconsciously until I had no reason left to go on, until everything and everyone had been removed from my life. I did not do this deliberately, as I had no idea what was causing this hurricane of trauma racing through my life. I built up a high pain threshold which hid everything else from sight.

Despite the damage I was doing, I kept trying to find a solution within the addiction. It was obvious to everyone else that it was destroying my life. However I was unaware of it for a very long time. With addiction, the destruction is rarely obvious to the addict when they are in the middle of it, and by the time it has become obvious to them, it is often too late.

The past guilt-ridden life with low self-worth was still lurking in my unconscious and without my conscious knowledge was orchestrating other problems, causing me to continually look for affirmation wherever it could be found.

When alcohol was removed from my life, this searching often led to other issues. I was taking uncalculated risks to try to recover a peaceful place, while continuously looking for acknowledgement.

So for many years it was total confusion as I chased down answers in the wrong areas outside of myself and not within myself. For many years my outer life was a direct picture of my inner life. It was dramatic and tragic as it followed the wrong clues.

So I had to find the source of my addiction and to find something that would bear real fruits of happiness in my life. I had been chasing the wrong solution to deliver the results I was looking for.

I had been trying to use a mind-altering substance to cure a MindBody symptom. My life was one of trauma until I found the source, the cause, and my shift from uneasiness to deliverance with real effects was exhilarating.

When I found the MindBody solution, my inner and outer life again became a copy of each other and became united and happy.

With my new MindBody awareness and acceptance, the void in my life is now filled, and the divided self has unified and I now have control of my mind and my body.

CHAPTER 4 A New Approach to Addiction

It is my belief that there is a new way to approach addictions like Alcoholism, Gambling, Drugs, Depression and Anorexia, which will resolve the currently unsolvable compulsive addictive life and which will provide a permanent solution.

In the case of the alcoholic this includes taking a drink of alcohol safely. For other addictions it will mean a new realisation and permanent recovery from the need for altering the mind unnaturally.

For people suffering from depression, they will realize that they are unconsciously addicted to their dark reservoir of repressed emotions. This is not a judgement, as people with addiction are usually unaware of their real problem. If they have not tried mind-altering substances themselves, they are often prescribed them by their medical services, leading to other forms of addiction.

The body and mind of the alcoholic or addict have become abnormal, sometimes from birth, more usually from the misuse of an addictive substance. In the case of brain damage inflicted through early life challenging situations, this damage can be reversed in natural ways without the need for a chemical prescription.

In the case of substance abuse, it is the mind-altered chemical process that creates the phenomena of craving in the addict. The mind altered perception of the end result prior to consuming the substance creates the mould, the cause, which once consumption takes place, approves the preconception, so that on withdrawal a need for replacement is the effect in every instance.

The abnormal becomes the normal from the beginning and has to be supported by continued use of mind-altering substances or actions.

The expectation of the result, like the law of attraction, creates the effect, prior to participation and when that perceived effect is not delivered by the drug, more of it is taken to reach it. The more that is taken, the more severe the withdrawal and the stronger the compulsive need there is to replenish again.

For many addicts this initial obsessional neediness which is never satisfied by a substance is replaced by the neediness for more of the same substance, during and after the consumption. This obsessional neediness finds expression in drink, drugs, food, sex, gambling, money, anorexia, etc., and often switches from one to the other as the addict tries to fill the gaping hole in the mind-altered false self.

For the majority of people, the enjoyable consumption of alcohol and spending money are just that and nothing else. For the addict, long before a decision to consume a drug, spend compulsively, eat or not eat, is taken, the intense craving for love, attention and approval, often subconscious and unknown to the seeker, manifests itself in many addictive ways and in the abuse of many substances, These same substances are used every day and normally by the majority of the population.

For the needy person who is trying to prove his worth, find love or approval, who is looking for someone or something to affirm him or her, the use of these substances amounts to the abnormal belief in their power to continually alter the mind on demand. This strong mind-altering affect, is first created by the user before use, something that does not occur with non addicts.

This belief is so strong; it creates a life-mould. So the mind becomes altered before, during and after the use of these substances and leaves one with a sense of excitement beforehand, a sense of achievement and belief in oneself during their presence and a real sense of loss as the substance-affect starts to leave the body.

It is this gradual withdrawal, this loss of belief in oneself, this feeling of being apart, this fear, this loss of worth, which creates the need for more of the substance (or in the case of anorexia, less of the substance). It creates a craving for continuous topping up or complete replacement by using or not using whatever the 'worth-creating' substance is.

In my own case, perhaps the loss of the natural state of bonding at childhood set up a life of neediness followed by a continual want to prove myself. This happened through no fault of my parents who gave to me the same love as they gave to my siblings. It was the lack in me; the void that craved more than was available or possible at the time.

It set in motion a life of acting on my nerves without any relaxation, a life where I always had the feeling of being apart from everything, a life where I was continually looking at myself from the outside in, as if I was someone else.

It created a life where I was afraid to be myself, because being myself was not accepted, and it was rejected when I was. My excessive emotional childhood neediness could not be filled by those around me, especially by my parents who had to spread their attention and love amongst twelve children.

I was self-obsessed from the day I was born. My addictive want to be the centre of the universe, to be an only child receiving all the love available, and the impossibility of its fulfilment, had a shocking affect on me as a little child.

Early on in my life, I mentally and sometimes physically left home and lived in the wilderness, finding solace on my own in the midst of bushes hidden in faraway fields.

I was not me anymore, I was acting the new me, whom I thought the world wanted me to be and I lost myself.

In the end I did not know who I was. It became frightening to be me, so I ran away at the first opportunity and never came back. Anytime I did come back, the world asked me; "Who are you?" really meaning "what are you good at?", "what have you achieved?", or "what worth have you?", and I had no answer.

Success was also a scary place to be and I soon forced failure again. The return to acting-out was like being home again. Being successful financially was part of that place they called awful, being bad and not being a good person, so it was better to sabotage and go back to another place, the mental place they impressed into my life plan that imprisoned me for many years of my life. A place where I could never fully accept love and often rejected it, as it was not from a human source and I knew no other.

The human source had never given it to me in the first place; they never had enough to give or go around. But the 'I of me', was always there, only no pathway was cleared yet to finding it. For me, the clearing of this pathway only came about after the almost complete destruction of myself.

This source, the 'I of me', is now obvious and has become the real source of my personal power, allowing others in and allowing me to be in control. The pathway is now clear.

CHAPTER 5 Being You now

For the addict, the mental state preceding the first drink or drug is the problem; it is not the drug per se that is the real problem. This mental state has to be corrected, altered to a new reality, to a new attitude, to the now, to the realization that you can change your own mind. This altered consciousness preceding the intake of the drug, programs the subconscious for the effect to happen when the drug is taken or given, depending on the type of substance.

It really is about who or what I am now and who or what do I want to become, and what do I believe will make me who or what I want to be at this moment in time.

What drink or drug will I use to be there now, to get there now, to be who or what now? The drink or drug works as long as it gets me from here to 'there', from whom or what I don't want to be, away from now, as quickly as possible.

If you don't take the drug now, wait a while; ask, what am I taking the drug for? Who do I want to be now, to be seen as now? What fears am I trying to avoid? Who do I want to impress with this drug-image of me now? Is it me I want to impress or accept? Is it others I want to impress or get acknowledged by?

Before taking the drug, ask what do I think is wrong with me now. Why do I need to be somewhere else or

34

someone else, anyone except me now? What do I really perceive is wrong with me, in this instant, at this time? Ask "what is going on in my life now?" and answer clearly and precisely.

Wait now, don't try to change now. See what it is really like not to act now. Be really you now.

Speeding away from you has consequences everywhere, with impatience, anger and frustration until another drug is found to change the moment for you, to change the mood, to alter you, so that you don't have to speed away from this new altered you. But once the drug leaves your system, so does the altered you and you are on the treadmill again, running away from you.

This is repeated endlessly. The drug-effect weakens and you need more and stronger doses to get you 'there', which is always getting further away from you, from who you really are. The real you is hidden behind the subconscious need to release the repressed feelings in your reservoir of strong emotions.

The solution is to stay as you are now. To do this you have to accept that you can talk to your brain, that you can truly heal yourself and your addictions. This is what you have been chasing all your life without knowing it; the real and only source of knowledge which was always there, but the pathway was hidden.

You are the only 'drug' you will ever need. Once you accept this fully, your life will be transformed in every area. Everything is in you and you are in everything.

You don't need to prove anything to anyone ever again. You are enough as you are. You are no longer alone. Through your thoughts you have been alone long enough. The separation is now over. The mind-altered false egoic self is gone once you stop and accept now as exactly the way it is meant to be at this moment.

You are you, here and now. You have the ability to change your mind, to change your body, to change your life. So next time you are truly looking for someone or something to change your life, look in the mirror, not in the bottle or in the drug.

As I did not fit the ideal image that I thought the world had for me, I was always speeding away from me, that scary monster that kept him away from me. Little did I know that this original me was okay and all versions since then were aberrations of this whole person.

I got to a stage in my early life where each aberration was developed individually as a fragment of the whole me, until knowing who I was, became impossible. I was cluttered fragments of many people trying to find their original home, their way home. I was willing to be like whoever I was with at the time, never allowing myself to truly be me.

Through acceptance of now being exactly the way it was meant to be, I got out of this mind alteration, this altered state of consciousness that became unconscious and was the cause that created every effect in my life.

So, you can break this glass mirror of your life that reflects the same bad story every time? You know now what the solution is that can stop the effect changing to another lethal obsession, just as the previous one is overcome. The answer is now, here and now, nothing else, when the fear of being you is overcome and accepted.

Many questions arose along my way to here. Very, very scary it seemed. What if you never reach you until you are old and ready to pass on? What if this is the way you are meant to live your life and no other. What if there is no answer, just you bumbling along. What if you are your parents? What if the only solution is being you?

What if your parents have passed away and you can never get that attention you so badly longed for all your life. Acceptance is the answer. It's time now to allow yourself to receive love and to give love back to others.

How are you going to fill that gaping lonely hole within you, who is going to hold you and say "I'm really proud of you, you are really good at what you do, I love you", as they wrap their arms around you and you feel really loved for the first time in your life and you don't have to prove anything to anyone ever again.

You always had the power to do this for yourself and you can now do it at will. You have to love yourself first.

For many, God is the only answer to that feeling of abandonment and detachment from life. For those people who believe in God, God will end the neediness and will always fill their wellbeing with the love they need, the love that they craved, that they used drink or other drugs to find. For others, taking responsibility for oneself is a more powerful and permanent source of power than searching for a God to believe in.

Addiction is a journey to finding yourself, if you survive it. For some it is a journey to finding God. For me it was a journey of education and knowledge, a journey to find my original self that held the power to control my mind and my body, a MindBody integration journey, powered by the 'I' of me.

The greatest challenge with your new view of life is that the person you think you are and that you have been fighting to keep and then fighting to get rid of, the person/ego that you blamed on your past, the ego you believed in and that was created by pain, is just a mind created impression and not who you really are. Because it is your familiar self, you continually resist any attempts to change it. In fact you regularly fight to defend it, to the point of aggressive points of view against those that don't match yours.

The solution to all the pain and constant looking back and looking forward is to wipe out the ego, this false mind-created you. Get rid of this by continually being in the present, through mindful meditation.

For some people it means coming into the presence of God, where there is no looking back or forward, just keeping the light of Presence on everything. This deletes the ego that was causing all the pain, the addiction and compulsion to drink and drugs, and the addiction to pleasing others and seeking approval.

The thought-made-me was the problem. I have changed this. Remember that you have absolute control over only one thing in your life, and that is your thoughts. This is very inspiring and reflects our true nature. With this power you can control your own destiny. If you fail to control your own mind, you will control nothing else. If you are allowing your thoughts to create and support the ego that drives your life, you will defend it to the end and live a false life based on misconceptions of who you really are.

This false life is frightening and leads to depression and addictions, where you fight to keep from losing this made-up identity, the identity which may have been made up initially to please your parents.

My life had become one of altered perceptions that were upheld for periods of time by substance abuse and other forms of escapism. Finding and realising my true powerful nature was the key to breaking free from my ego, or false self.

Through your true nature you can stop being a control freak, live in the present, switch off the past and the future and work with the self that is here and now. This is who you are.

You are not a collection of past experiences or future dreams. You are who you are now without a past or future. In this moment you are all you ever wanted to be, which is present in your life, or in the Presence.

When you get this right everything else is illuminated by it and the possibilities are endless. There are no thought-made ego barriers preventing your success. The ego is gone when you are in this state and you are whole.

The length of time you can stay in this state of Presence, this Now, determines the length of time that the allergic addictions have no power over you. They have no affect on you in the now and never will have.

Addiction affects you when your mind-made false egoic self, no matter what personal trauma or loss created it originally, compulsively switches from past to future to past to future, never finding you in the present.

You stumble around in the dark past looking for a new future, always missing the target. It is time to stop looking in the dark and switch on the light of the present, the Presence.

CHAPTER 6 The Present

The beginning of total recovery from addiction is the realisation that you are not the addict; your false mind-made self is. When you are in present moment awareness you can drink and stop at any time. The opposite is true when your MindBody state is doing the drinking, it needs constant refreshing to remain in the same drink induced state, otherwise, if you pause for a while, it starts to panic and gets frightened and the phenomena of craving is activated.

As the withdrawal starts, the false mind-made self is afraid of losing its new identity, that new state that taking a drink has created. It is the same for addicts when drink is not involved, the false self is constantly fighting to survive, always looking back or looking forward, never in the present, on edge, constantly trying to fit in and people-please, so that eventually you have no idea who you really are.

Compulsion and addiction do not live in present moment awareness. They are created by the belief and acceptance of the false mind-made egoic self and sustained by continuous efforts to save this self from annihilation, from dying, from being proven wrong.

It is in the new acceptance of the real you and the elimination of the false you, that allows normality to exist in your life, probably for the first time ever. The false self is so engrained, sometimes through early trauma that it will fight to the bitter end to remain you, as it sees you.

41

The battle you have is simpler than you think. You don't need to analyze the past (the dark) to move on, to find the real you. All you need to do is to switch on the light of the present and stay in the present light awareness. The past disappears into the light.

Fighting the past is not the answer, it is the problem and helps the false egoic self to continually survive and recreate itself, keeping you stuck forever. The ego will keep creating and sustaining new pasts if you focus on it, in a never-ending cycle.

The answer is switching on the light and the dark disappears and your every-moment presence ensures that no new pasts are created. You live in the now.

As long as you identify with your mind and not the present moment, the false egoic self ru(i)ns your life and you are constantly either looking backwards for solutions or forwards in fear. You are not living in the present, the real world. The ego is insecure and feels constantly under threat, even when the person looks confident on the outside.

It is a constant balancing act which can manifest in many ways including constantly trying to prove yourself, people-pleasing and never knowing who you truly are. In the false egoic mind-created self you constantly try to adjust to everyone else rather than ruffle the feathers of this false self. You have no voice and when you do, it comes across as aggressive or defensive.

The ego fights to survive and makes you think it is you, so you live in constant fear, fear of being found out, of not being good enough. This fear is often reflected in your failures, in your inability to let go and go forward with any burning desire to succeed. The fear often arises just as it looks like you might be successful and sabotages your success.

The constant need for approval and affirmation are daily companions in your life. When you find your identity in being, in the present or in the Presence, this egoic false self disappears along with all its psychotic compulsions. The light of awareness has been switched on and envelopes your whole life.

Your Self, your identity is now the present, no looking back or forward except for practical reasons. Your Self exists now. It does not exist anywhere else. This light of Presence needs to be kept on; otherwise you will slip back into your past.

The dark false egoic self needs constant reassurance, constant escapes and addictive compulsions for it to survive.

Absolutely nothing addictive will happen when you are fully in the present, in the Presence, no matter what mind altering substance you take, because you are not identifying your Self with your mind any more.

This is the key. This is the solution to total recovery. It is foolproof. As your true Self exists only in the present and is fine, you have no 'need' to alter or defend your mind-identified self anymore and you are not taking a drug to alter your mind anymore.

The steps to realization and living in the Presence need not take years of pain. There is no requirement for penance, fasting or suffering. You have had enough of that already and it doesn't solve anything. When the false self is gone, there is nothing to fight, nothing to try to change.

Compulsion arises from trying to get rid of the false self using a drug followed by the fight back from the ego which fights to prevent any change to it.

It is a monster that when dampened by drug use, seems to grow larger when the drug withdraws and the inner you screams for you to return to this escape area, to another mind altered self, so you are jumping from one mind-altered self to another mind(drug) altered self and your True self is unknown.

With active addiction, more and more mind altering is needed until it kills you in the end.

CHAPTER 7 A Mind Need

My subconscious need for affirmation became the conscious addiction to the continuous want for an unattainable wellbeing. This wellbeing was sought by the ingestion of alcohol and other mind-altering substances.

The subconscious was made whole for a time by this conscious ingestion until the whole became a hole as the substance withdrew from the body. The neediness was then retriggered and set the addiction in motion all over again.

I now know that this neediness can never be filled by physical means and the victim / addict is often driven to despair, physically, then mentally, trying to satisfy this need.

Satisfaction only comes through realization that this need has no physical fulfilment. Fulfilment only comes through a realization or awareness of its MindBody reality, and then it disappears, is no longer there. The light of awareness needs to be shone if the neediness ever makes itself known again.

Addiction was always a compulsion to fill a mind gap, to fill a mind need, to fulfil an emotional need, to fill a life need. It was like trying to catch the wind. It was never available to be caught, as only MindBody awareness made it accessible, and awareness was missing.

Once awareness made it accessible and the realization that it was a subconscious need, then and only then could it be transformed into a non-need and made right, so that alcohol and other substances were no longer needed as there was no hole to fill and the being became whole through awareness.

The solution comes through accepting that the subconscious neediness was the trigger for physical craving. The subconscious neediness is never satisfied, as it is trying to satisfy a non-conscious reality. It can however be got rid of through awareness.

MindBody awareness is the light which clears away this dark part of your life. The solution to any addiction is going back to the 'Being' of being human and realizing its need for affirmation and acceptance, as the human part of being is led to look for a physical response.

In the addict, the closest to satisfaction of this need arises after the first few drinks or drugs are taken by the addict. A near state of 'bliss' is reached. This state does not occur in the non-addict. For the addict, this state of bliss quickly evaporates and more alcohol is consumed and drunkenness sets in.

The victim/addict has to drink more to try to get back to that state of bliss again, which is impossible, because the early blissful state only arrives during the first few drinks and the effect of the drink cannot be reversed when in the process of drinking.

So the chase begins, with the victim/addict chasing an impossible dream, a need that was moved from the subconscious to the conscious and back again, through ingestion of a mind altering substance.

For non-addicts the subconscious neediness never existed in the first place and therefore the ingestion of alcohol is always a physical act with no expected emotional, mental or subconscious attachment and no overwhelming feeling of filling a void through ingestion of the substance.

The normal person is not aware of a subconscious need and does not need to satisfy one. Whereas the addict is subconsciously always aware of a neediness, an emptiness, something missing, a feeling of low self-worth, low self esteem, a lacking that needs something to fill it.

So the subconscious neediness is the original disease, the addiction. This is then acted out on the physical plane with no let up, because there is no physical solution!

MindBody awareness is the cure. Drinking socially then becomes a purely physical act with no expected solutions to be solved, only nice physical effects, that are not craved for or needed, but are a bonus when they happen. They are an added benefit and not the primary reason for taking the drink.

So when the addict stops drinking, through spiritual or other means (the second birth), the subconscious neediness will find other outlets, other ways of being affirmed through other activities, or substances.

The subconscious will still need to fill its needy hole. It will become compulsive and go to the ends of the earth to find satisfaction for its subconscious unease which will manifest in physical disease if it is not expressed outwardly, or in addiction if it is.

The physical activities or substances will never satisfy the subconscious as it doesn't know what it is trying to satisfy – it is only a fleeting feeling that it chases, so we move from one addiction to another, one compulsion to another. We stop one and take up another, unless we reach the MindBody realization of what is going on.

The 'willing to believe' in AA stopped my drinking, but it did not stop the subconscious unease, which could be recreated physically anytime with only one drink. The drink-effect attaches itself to the subconscious need for affirmation and continues to try to satisfy this subconscious craving for attention, sometimes until the physical person is dead.

In AA the unease remains in the subconscious and is only arrested one day at a time through dependence on a higher power and attending AA meetings where the person's achievement in staying sober is continually affirmed.

For many the 'belief' or 'higher power' is the AA meeting and both work equally well in arresting the addiction at work in the conscious or physical plane. As long as one distracts the subconscious from its neediness, all is okay. But the disease remains in the subconscious and can be activated at any time when destruction of the original disease has not happened.

The cure (the third birth) is acceptance of the MindBody creation of the addiction as a diversion or self-safety valve and then to look at, release and remove the power from these repressed emotions. Awareness is the solution.

Other addictions like drugs, sex and gambling all can be cured in a similar way, by looking at the low self-worth of the subconscious, accepting it for what it is and giving it the light of MindBody education, knowledge and awareness, and then one will see that there is no neediness to satisfy.

In relation to other addiction issues, the feeling of low self esteem can give you a life ridden with guilt, a feeling of not being good enough, a feeling of dis-ease. Other addictions can often take centre stage, when a previous one is removed from the addict's life.

I do not need any more self-help training or any more life lessons. I have learned the biggest lesson and do not need to have another birth in order to realize my subconscious unease that manifested in chronic alcoholism.

It is healed now. The chain is broken, now I can get on with my life and have a drink safely whenever I like.

Lack of self worth and the unconscious reservoir of trauma, began the process of my addiction, of using drink to feel good, and looking for approval all the time.

In AA when the need for self worth and drink is replaced by God or a Higher Power, the need is filled, but other 'needs' arise and need to be handed over as well. It's an ongoing process that has no end unless one reaches MindBody awareness and solves the subconscious self worth issues and dis-eases.

This is the self worth issue that needs continuous approval and affirmation by self and others, so the AA meetings work well to keep one away from drink. However, AA is of no value if you would like to drink socially again.

When I drank, I drank into my subconscious, to fill a need, the whole had a hole. Now drink will only go to the conscious and will not be re-needed to fill a subconscious void, as it doesn't exist anymore.

In the beginning, when I took a drink I used it to become the person I thought I should be. When I stopped drinking and went to AA meetings I became the person I always was; still with an unease, a void or hole to be filled.

This was a needy sensitive person, a soul searcher, a person looking for answers, a person with a void in their lives, who could no longer hide in compulsive drinking, or in enforced abstinence.

When alcohol was removed from my life, the MindBody system produced chronic physical pain as the next diversion from my repressed emotions.

So before drinking again, there is a need for a period of adjustment, or acceptance of this new person, this stranger. A period of abstinence from alcohol is required, where emotional and physical recovery is followed by a new awareness and perception of the subconscious, the place where all this neediness, unease and disease began.

You can drink safely when you say you can. Like alcoholics at a religious service, you can drink the wine safely, because you say you can, and you believe you can. It is the same with a bottle of wine from the Off Licence. When you have this same belief in your true self, your true power, you can create, be, do and achieve anything. You can also take a drink safely and enjoy every drop of it.

CHAPTER 8 Over The Influence

Alcoholism, like chronic pain, depression, gambling, debting and drug addiction can be cured and cured permanently, allowing the sufferer to drink socially. This might be shocking and scary for some people attending AA meetings.

I was clinically diagnosed as suffering from chronic alcoholism and have been off drink, continuously sober and attending AA meeting for over 30 years.

I had all the classic symptoms of chronic alcoholism from an early age; obsession, craving, compulsion, never able to stop after the first drink, hangovers, never able to get enough alcohol, blackouts, 'geographicals', delirium tremens, alcoholic convulsions, cures in the morning, missing work, continuous medical certificates, regular admissions to General and Mental hospitals, rehab programs, crashes, injuries, debt, sick and depressed after many years of torture. I was addicted to drink since my early teens.

Following the discovery of my true self and the formation of Over the Influence (OTI), I am now able to drink like any social drinker. I now know that like chronic pain, alcoholism can be cured permanently, without the need for psychotherapy, drugs, abstinence or surgery. You can drink socially again, even if you were alcoholic from day one and never drank socially in the first place!

In meetings of Over the Influence (OTI) we speak about who we really are with or without a drink. Our new power for living is in us and we live in the question, not the answer. The answer is provided by our being. We don't need drink to open up to our fellow members.

If we are having a drink we can feel safe among like-minded people. We can also feel comfortable having a drink in any other situation as it has now become just another part of our life, and not all of our life, like it used to be. Alcohol is not the problem, so abstinence is not the solution. You are the problem and you are the solution.

Up to now, the 'phenomena of craving' which Bill Wilson describes so well, was always present in the subconscious, with or without alcohol. It will only become absent with or without alcohol, when the OTI answer is accepted.

To get started you need to look at what alcohol means to you and meant to you from day one. It doesn't matter whether alcohol was used in your house as an escape from the worries of the world or whether your parents drank socially or never drank.

In relation to genetic links to alcoholism it would be more accurate to examine the epigenetic transfer of personality. Alcohol was the drug of choice for many in previous generations also. Where this was not a factor in previous generations, epigenetic factors often created the addictive conditions for alcoholism to grow.

Chemically many of us have a disposition to drink more than others, however for this to progress to alcoholism or chronic alcoholism as in my case really depends on your MindBody interaction and your reservoir of strong emotions.

Alcoholism is dependence on alcohol at its most basic. For the majority of alcoholics, some areas of their life are seriously affected by their drinking. With chronic alcoholism you have no other life; every area of your life is affected by excessive consumption of alcohol.

Up to now it was generally accepted that there was no cure for alcoholism. Abstinence was seen as the only solution and people who took a drink again usually died by suicide, a serious accident or ended up permanently incarcerated in a mental asylum. Why is this?

The answer is simple, yet it is the most complicated way of looking at this for some people. Alcohol is not the problem and never has been the problem, the problem is what alcohol means or meant to us, what meaning we attached to it.

For the majority of people, alcohol is not used to balance any inadequacies they have in their lives. For addicts, once they get started on that balancing act it is very difficult to turn back and the results are catastrophic for ourselves and those around us.

The 'fixing' need becomes ever greater as we progress and the quantity needed to get back to where we started, gets bigger. We never really get back to the little discomforts that we thought we needed to use alcohol for. These are continually replaced by bigger discomforts and the consumption of alcohol goes up every time to try to reach 'down' to the earlier place, so that we can move 'up' to a better place.

What most addicts never realise is that nearly everyone has some discomfort and accepts it as part of life. Addicts can rarely accept this and always want a four legged stool of a life, one that is fully balanced all the time. This is not reality as mostly everyone gets out of balance at some time in their lives. Alcoholics are continually running after shadows trying to find the missing leg.

Let's get off the fence. AA has saved my life and the lives of countless others as well. Without it I would have died over 30 years ago. It 'arrested' my compulsive drinking through complete abstinence and gave me back a new life that I had never experienced before. Yet I could never take a drink again safely I was told.

In my family, drink was consumed in large amounts, yet no one ever got addicted like I did. I was the only one who could not stop when I took a drink. Why was this?

I went to the pub for alcohol first, and for socializing second. My family went to the pub for a chat, meet friends, have a few drinks and a good time. They took alcohol as they were doing this. Drink was not attached to identification of their Self. Alcohol was not the main object of their visit to the pub, and even when it was, it was not the total focus of their mind. They were not using it to get to another place, away from where they were in their mind.

They had discomforts, irritations, annoyances, yet they accepted them as part of life. They had a three legged stool of a life; sometimes it was great, sometimes it was pretty bad, most times it simply was okay, no major ups or downs. They did not need to prove anything or do anything special to get along in life. They fitted in to the way things were. When they wanted to clean the slate and forget, they talked it out with a friend or spouse, just as they did with good news. It was no big deal. It was just life.

For people who drift into dependence on alcohol, the alcohol becomes life and life becomes alcohol. The object of their desire is alcohol and it must be satisfied first before other pleasures are partaken. Alcohol is their saviour from an 'ordinary' life which they cannot accept and find continually discomforting.

For the alcoholic, alcohol 'saves' and 'saves' and 'saves' and then kills. Ordinary discomforts are not allowed for the alcoholic. A continuous feeling of good form is required or else they feel the attraction or compulsion for their friend alcohol.

The over-use of alcohol to attain 'normality' is a catch twenty two situation, where the excesses lead to bad health and other personal and mental problems which are continually increased by the over consumption.

What is the solution? Obviously it is necessary to stop for a while to take a look at your situation and allow yourself to recover physically and mentally. It is then necessary to accept the awareness that life is okay, and is exactly as it is meant to be right now. It doesn't have to be good all the time. It doesn't have to be full-on-joy twenty four hours a day.

Ask your social drinking neighbour and you'll see that they have plenty of ups and downs. They don't need a four legged stool of a life, when a three legged one will do most of the time.

Remember you can drink safely now, not yesterday, not tomorrow, but now. You can do everything you want now. Your mind now is capable of safely drinking. Once you leave now and your drinking is in tomorrow or yesterday, you are doomed to the obsessive and addictive compulsion, to return to where you always were.

Your drinking is just a symptom of your MindBody need to escape from now, from you, and a compulsive desire to create a new you through a physical substance or the absence of a physical substance as in anorexia.

Your compulsive need to be not you, creates a new entity (the addiction), giving the drug of choice a new power, a new being, that holds, in your mind, the answer to your problems.

In some cases you will deliberately try to create this affect, when not taking any drug, by trying not to be you, and mask your true self through various outward actions and expressions, that you think others think are you. You can get caught up in this circus act and lose yourself completely, even without taking a drug.

I could have taken the easy road, but I didn't know where it was. I was on a road that was going around in circles, going back to the dark, looking for answers in the past and ending up in the same place every time, neither in the past, present or future, in limbo waiting for life to begin or end and sometimes deliberately trying to end it.

Then creating a false self and trying to live with it and creating character defects to survive the life it gave me.

Now I am in the MindBody knowledge, the light. The dark is gone. There is no past and the future I want is a seed planted, grown and nourished in the present.

The facts are that life is not easy all the time for everyone else. Most people have to go through awkward moments to arrive at a place of relaxation. The stool does not always have to be balanced. Sometimes one leg is wobbly for a while. That is human nature.

To strive obsessively to have everything in balance all the time is the cause of many problems. Let go and allow yourself to fall down some times. Have a good circle of friends that will hold you up and support you when you need it. Go to Over the Influence (OTI) meetings, have a few beers and share with like-minded people.

Have someone you can share everything with, or if not, make sure that you can share openly with many close friends, sharing all your secret bits with many different people if necessary.

CHAPTER 9 You are the Solution

Acquiring and retaining happiness comes from within. The solution to fear of something, whether it's dancing or meeting people is to confront the fear by learning the skills in baby steps, so that you can move beyond that fear.

Often behind our greatest fear lies our greatest treasure. Using a mind altering substance to rid yourself of the fear will continually divert you from facing it and finding your treasure, which is often within the fear.

When you use a substance (or non substance as in the case of anorexia) as a solution to something you fear, whether the fear is based in reality or not, the substance might work for a short time and cause your mind to focus on it instead of the fear, but the substance itself then becomes the problem as its initial effect wears off and the original fears still remain and become more frightening because the substance is no longer hiding them.

A happy life is an inside job, an awareness and transformation process for many of us, that takes time, and something many of us refuse to do until we are on our knees for the thousandth time, asking " Why Me"?.

The resulting good feeling from overcoming your fears and changing your life naturally, is a million times better than any initial buzz you might get from trying to numb your fears with a mind altering substance.

To eventually succeed you have to become okay with feeling uncomfortable, trying and failing a few times before you reach your goal.

Once you understand and accept the MindBody source of your addiction, and accept that you are powerful, more powerful than you ever imagined, you can then drink any alcoholic beverage without having the phenomenon of craving and without becoming addicted again.

The first time I realised this was one day I went to a Service in a Protestant church to see what a Protestant service was like. I was offered Communion in bread and wine and I decided there and then that if I truly believed what I am saying in this book, that the wine was non-addictive, then it would not have any effect on me. So I drank it and it had no addictive effect on me. It did not set up any craving for more.

Both I and alcohol can survive and enjoy each other when I have a right relationship with my true self and a true understanding of the MindBody source of my original unease that led to addiction.

I was always aware, that despite being part of a large family, that no other members of my family were addicted to alcohol. We all lived in the same epigenetic environment, the same house, went through mostly the same experiences. None of the other members of my family had a passion to leave home like I did either.

My addiction was in me. It was not in them. Maybe it was there from my womb experience, when I was born, or from my early childhood. It doesn't really matter, once I know that I can change my addictive nature with this new MindBody education, knowledge, understanding and power.

The survival tools I used as a child became my tormentor as they grew into my identity. What I thought then was the 'I' of me, was a false mind made self, which had no core, no substance and wavered at the whims of those around me. It was trying to fit in and look good with everyone, and constantly seeking approval.

In my early years, up to age 28, alcohol was my power, my mind, my God. Then in AA, God became my alcohol. Then with my new MindBody knowledge 'I' became my power and my MindBody integration knowledge cured my addiction for good. Then alcohol became just another drink. Then my True self emerged and consciousness provided everything I needed, every time I let it.

Alcohol was never the problem, I was. So I was the solution, not abstinence. However, to realize this you may need to be abstinent for a period of time.

So don't create your life on what is not real or true. Don't buy into lies about what a true life is. It's what we think we can't have that becomes valuable. Once you realize that you can have anything you want, it doesn't matter that much anymore.

Remember, you are the problem, not drink or drugs or any other mind altering addiction, and if you are still looking for that one person who can change your life, all you need to do is take a look in a mirror. You are the only one in the universe that knows everything about you and your life. You are the only one that is powerful enough to stop you changing. To change, you need to be willing to receive. The true I of you is the only one powerful enough to start changing you, now.

To the questions of your life, you are the only answer. To the problems of your life, you are the only solution. If your life is filled with stress and anger, look at what your self-worth is based on. Is it based on objects, ideas and the approval of others? Base it on your true self, which is conscious awareness of the 'I' of you, and it will fill your life with true and lasting power.

CHAPTER 10 Healthy Minded

The healthy minded need only be born once, physically and emotionally. The sick souls like me, born with a divided self, must be born twice and often three times, in order to find happiness.

The second birth usually takes place following prolonged trauma in our lives, when we seek a new way of living and are forced to consider that 'our' way alone, is not the answer.

For us divided souls, the spiritual and the natural are at odds, and we must lose or let go of one before we can participate in the other.

Unfortunately for many people during active addiction, losing one's life often means taking one's life, as I tried to do many times. This is not what I mean here. We lose our old way of doing things, our old life, as we become willing to accept a new way. We start to move away from the pure natural to the emotional and spiritual, thereby integrating both.

Divided souls who are not aware of their divided self and do not know how to resolve and integrate it, often end up suffering mental illness and despair, often ending in suicide.

Until MindBody integration or willingness to accept this new way of thinking happens, the world appears a double sided and confusing mystery.

Divided souls need this second birth, a rebirth which is not necessary for those healthy souls who have an integrated emotional, spiritual and natural life from birth, something which most people have and are unaware of.

The healthy minded have their emotional, spiritual and natural aspects integrated from birth and do not need to go through this process which can be extremely harrowing for those of us who have experienced it and come out the other side. Many do not make it through.

Coming to believe in yourself as the greatest power you have is the solution to a divided self, the divided self that has caused disease and addiction in your life.

You don't need to believe at the start, you only need to become willing to believe. This power can be personal to you and for some it might be part of their religious beliefs. Whatever it is for you, it is for you. It is the first and most powerful method of recovery from the divided self. This divided self leads to depression, suicidal thoughts, addictions and other emotional traumas.

Your new MindBody power can be found through meditation, through prayer, or just through a willingness to believe. You can name this power God or whatever you like, but the concept you are after, is belief in the loving presence of a power that has all the attributes of God, and only the good God-attributes that have been portrayed by all the major peaceful religions and mystical organisations around the world.

To start the healing process, become willing to believe that you have control, that you are no longer powerless over alcohol or any other addiction.

Daily meditation has been proven to prolong and make permanent, the acceptance of your MindBody integration power in your life. You can heal your life and addictions, no matter what traumas you may have experienced throughout your life.

It has been proven without any shadow of doubt, by neuroscientists, using MRI scanning during meditation and prayer, with monks, nuns, meditation groups, mystics, beginners and advanced meditators, believer and non-believers, that meditation, a belief in God or any other spiritual practice, enhances your brains functionality and makes physical changes in your neural circuitry, giving long term benefits.

We won't get into the anatomy of the brain here or the various regions of the brain that switch on or off during meditation or prayer as there are many good books out there outlining this in great detail. It is only necessary to become willing, or to fake it till you make it, to get started on this brain enhancement process. It will take time.

You can change your life and your family tree. You don't have to be stuck in the fear cycles that you created up to now or that were created for you when you were young and vulnerable.

Your brain will eventually catch up and start to believe in your new self talk, and your life will change and you will always have your MindBody power available to you to get you through any rough times. This is not a cop out. It is a scientifically proven way of changing the neural circuitry in your brain for the better. You can do this as a believer or non-believer; it doesn't matter to your brain.

Complete and absolute honesty with yourself is important when you start to look at the source of addiction in your life. Doing it any other way brings continuous lessons to learn until you accept honesty in every area of your life as the only way to live this new life.

Being true to yourself means accessing your true self, that which is pure consciousness, which existed before your physical body and will exist after your physical body. This conscious self becomes tainted when you attach it to mind images and cause it to block your conscience.

Your conscious self is always good, non-addicted, loving and joyful, so reach back to it and find this place and remain there. It will attract only good into your life.

Once you accept and practice this you will see and experience a new life, you will be reborn. You will start being honest with yourself and others. You cannot fool yourself or others and get away with it. This is my painful experience. Life will keep sending you challenges until you accept this rebirth into a second truthful honest existence.

Acceptance of this is the first step in the new life and practice keeps it alive, so that all new challenges bring you forward to greater true and long lasting joy. The truth, your True self, will set you free.

CHAPTER 11 Depression

Depression usually accompanies active addicts on their journey to despair. Depression is also a disease in its own right and people with depression may not have addiction problems. But people with addiction problems are nearly always depressed.

Depression can be permanently eradicated from the victim's life through use and acceptance of this same MindBody integration knowledge and by using the OTI recovery program, whether you have addiction problems or not.

In MindBody parlance, depression is the unconscious addiction to despair and misery. This is not a judgment, as the person suffering from depression is usually unaware that the creation of depression is a similar process to that of the creation of MindBody pain or addiction.

Like addiction, depression is unconsciously created as a diversion mechanism and functions in the same way as alcohol addiction or chronic pain diversion symptoms.

In the case of depression, power is given to the condition instead of to a substance.

Undesirable emotions repressed for many years can influence both our physical and emotional wellbeing when they are being withheld from the conscious mind.

Why depression is there, is irrelevant. You only need to switch on the light of awareness today and move on from where you are now. The switch that brings you back to addiction or depression can be chemical, emotional or physical. The switch that brings you out of it turns on a new light in your life. So stop wallowing in the dark, the past and moping around without a torch. Switch on the MindBody awareness light.

How do you find the torch to switch on the light? The Light is created through your awareness of your true self, the presence in your life and the torch is your willingness to believe in this presence, this MindBody integration that truly works.

Whatever you call this belief is irrelevant, whether it is called God, Spirituality, Allah or Buddha does not matter. All that matters is that you connect with the 'I' of you; that internal spiritual and emotional part of you. If you use meditation to do this, it will change the neural circuitry in your brain to one of positive optimism and belief in yourself. This has been proven beyond doubt by many neuro-scientific tests over the last twenty years.

You don't have to be connected with any religious organisation to reach this state. You can link it to your religion if you wish and it may have a greater impact for you.

You can connect with your emotional and spiritual side in many ways and meditation is only one of them. Once you have the willingness to believe, you then have the tools to shine the MindBody integration knowledge on the present, to illuminate and destroy the dark (the past). The past has no power in your life once you switch on this Light.

You cannot find answers in the Past. You can only change your future from the present.

What causes the stress, the depression, the addiction in your life, is trying to live in the future while focusing and dwelling in the past, in the dark.

For the Illuminated, the past does not exist, only the present. The present well lived, is the creator of your future. The future is in your present.

When MindBody illumination occurs, the present is the seed that grows daily into the future you choose today. So you have a choice of how your life will unfold. You need to first accept today as exactly how you are meant to feel today, as it's meant to be.

You created what is in your life today, maybe not deliberately but it has resulted from the seeds you planted in your mind. Nothing is accidental in your thoughts, they are governed by you and you have the power to think differently about what is going on in your life.

You have control, and once you realise this, you can change everything. Your peace of mind is not dependant on what you have, unless what you have defines who you think you are.

Your peace of mind is a daily thing, based always on acceptance of the light in your life, based always on acceptance that the dark (the past) is now gone. Darkness cannot survive in the light, try it!

Can you find a torch to shine darkness on a sunny day? Darkness is the absence of light and has no power of itself. It cannot darken the Light unless you live in the past. Light is acceptance of presence, not the absence of dark. In the presence there is no dark, only light.

Living in the present today, gives a present that is full, whole and needs nothing else to define it. Defining your present by constant reference to the past, colours every day of your life with a dark shadow that you have invited into your life.

Why is it that people are constantly going back to the past in counselling and psychotherapy? Why is that once they have finished years of this 'darkness therapy' they go back again and again and seek another past (dark) to live in.

Why does the past define them? Why are they afraid of the Light and not of the Dark? Because it allows them to postpone living in the present, in the Presence.

The Dark is no longer with us when the light is switched on. The Light cannot be put out by the Dark when you accept MindBody illumination and carry your presence awareness torch with you. This torch can be shone into and illuminate every corner of your life.

You have the choice to turn the switch on (the Presence) or off (dark past). Focusing on the present will change your brain circuitry. See the present as hope, as love as joy. Even if you only focus on this for half an hour a day it will start to rewire your brain so that it sees the Light.

Belief and acceptance of this new MindBody integration knowledge, and your faith-state or prayer-state creates an inflow of positive energy. Your life, once only a life of division, struggle and addiction, now becomes unified as you surrender your lower self and your personal centre to this higher force.

Spiritual strength will increase and a new life will open up to you. There was something 'wrong' with you before and now it has been righted. You are saved from the 'wrongness' by making proper connection with your higher self and surrendering your will or lower self.

Once you make a start to accept this wrongness, you immediately will begin to move beyond it and will experience the first signs of serenity and peace. You will begin to see and feel the better part of you once you become willing to believe in a power greater than your lower self.

You will then slowly begin to accept your real being as the germinal part of your higher self. You will become more conscious of this higher power, this higher part of yourself and you can work with it in practical ways in your life. Get on board and save yourself. All your lower being has brought to you is struggle and despair.

Your divided self and life of struggle were a preparation for acceptance of this fact. For us of this disposition, there is no other or better way if we are to survive and live a life of happiness. We have to change our personal centre of self-will and surrender our lower self and accept the help of a higher self, or the 'I' of us, into our lives.

When you throw yourself into this, your life will take on a new meaning and a new energy that it never had before. This sense of union with a power within us is not merely apparent, but literally true as we become more in contact with all the faculties of our subconscious which makes this connection possible. This unseen force or power produces real effects in your world.

God is the usual name given by Christians for this supreme reality, this higher power. This book is not connected to any religious sect or organisation so you can just call it your true self, higher power or a name that describes its power best for you. This power is real and produces real practical effects in your life. Your life will take a turn for the better or the worse in proportion to your connection to this limitless power.

People of a religious or spiritual disposition, often give up the feeling of personal responsibility, letting go their hold and resigning the care of their destiny to higher powers and become generally indifferent as to what becomes of it all.

For me, with this new MindBody knowledge it is important to take personal control of your own life, and give up the habit of always relying on an external source. When you find your true self, you will give your private compulsive self a rest.

Instead of pursuing vague ideals, become the partaker of this infinite and abundant life. Become the creator and manifestor of your new positive thought-made life.

My early years of swallowing and repressing rage were followed by active addiction. Then abstinence from the addictive substance resulted in chronic pain, released throughout my body by the undesirable unresolved repressed emotions, until finally, acceptance, awareness and belief in my MindBody integration power, led to the final cure.

CHAPTER 12 Repression

Physical, emotional or sexual abuse as a child can often be the starting point for the repression of rage, anger and other strong emotions. These stressors instil a very low level of self-esteem in a child, leading to perfectionism and people-pleasing throughout their lives.

For much of my life I felt frightened, abandoned, insecure, introverted, desperately looking for other's approval and never happy with my own successes, which were often significant. I blame no one for the addicted being I became or how my life turned out; it was in me and I had to experience it. To heal I had to forgive myself and others in order to prevent their influence from dominating my relationships.

Repression of emotions was a safety mechanism I used. It was mostly done unconsciously, to prevent these undesirable and frightening emotions from escaping into my consciousness.

These strong emotions often lay dormant until other life stressors eventually overflowed my repressed reservoir and activated these emotions into my body through addiction, depression and physical pain.

As well as causing pain in many parts of my body, swallowing and repressing strong emotions led to ulcers, allergies and depression. When I stopped drinking alcohol, the emotions that alcohol was helping to repress and divert attention from, began to surface.

As a result of my early years experience I became self sufficient too young. Over time, I had to learn to treat my inner child, the way I treat my own children, i.e. with love and understanding.

My inner child's personality was still immature, a young child's personality, that was trying to live in an adult world, in an adult body. I had to stop letting the little child make decisions in my life.

For years I had been unable to verbalize my pain and used the only language I knew, which was my body or my unconscious mind. I remember someone saying to me that I was like a coiled spring, ready to explode.

Through AA I was able to release some of this pain in a safe environment and began to realize that I was not alone in feeling the way I did. However, much deeper rage began to surface and cause severe physical pain in many parts of my body.

The pain in my lower back became so intense at one stage that I was referred for surgery. Shortly before surgery, I completely healed my back pain with MindBody integration knowledge, and I did not require surgery or any other medical intervention.

I have healed many other severe debilitating conditions using this treatment model ever since then.

Like physical pain and depression, alcoholism was just another symptom or side effect of my repressed reservoir of emotional pain. The addiction was created unconsciously as a diversion to prevent strong repressed emotions from becoming conscious.

When the addiction was 'arrested one day at a time' in AA, physical pain became the next diversion mechanism. If medication was used to mask this diversion, many other forms of diversion could have taken place; like other addictions, depression, anorexia etc. However I was fortunate not to use any mind altering medication and to discover the MindBody process that precipitated these diversions and was able to prevent this ongoing cycle of physical pain and addiction and to cure both of them, naturally.

So I have overcome my physical pain and overcome my addiction. My pain bordering on depression at times and my addiction, were all symptoms of the underlying repressed emotions that I had stored since childhood.

Addiction and pain were created, without my conscious knowledge, as a diversion to prevent my repressed trauma from becoming conscious.

In the Western world today chronic physical pain and addiction is rampant and so is emotional pain like depression. Many of these physical and emotional conditions lead to suicidal states. In many countries suicide has now become the biggest killer of men under fifty.

My addiction to alcohol happened because it was the most available drug to divert exposure from my underlying repressed emotions. Had I been exposed to other drugs, I would have taken them also, and they would have had the same effect. I would have become addicted to them, addicted to their ability to hide my true feelings.

Later in life when I'd stopped drinking for many years and started to experience severe physical pain throughout my body, I began to realise that both the addiction and the pain were just different facets of each other, different sides of the same coin.

I now know that I have control over whether I'm addicted or not. I also know that I have control over my physical and emotional pain.

I've been able to completely heal my physical pain using my mind and the knowledge of the source of my pain. I have also been able to heal the source of my addiction.

Addiction is no longer necessary. Its purpose has been exposed. The diversion is no longer needed.

Despite living without alcohol for over 30 years I still had issues that came up, resulting from the deep repressed emotions that were continually adding to my reservoir of rage. I lived a life of white-knuckle survival in AA, repressing my real desires, one of which was to drink socially.

Many people have saved their lives by stopping drinking. This was my experience. If I had not stopped drinking when I did, I have no doubt but that I would not be alive today. So I'm not saying that staying sober in Alcoholics Anonymous is a negative thing, I'm saying that there is a way that alcoholics can drink safely and socially once they understand the MindBody source of their addiction and accept the source as the cause that created the effect, which is the addiction, the pain or the addicted personality.

Like recovery from physical pain through MindBody knowledge, it is not necessary to remove or to psychoanalyse your trauma or strong emotions, to get rid of the addiction. It is only necessary to understand and acknowledge these repressed emotions as the first and only cause of your addiction.

The addiction and pain is created to divert conscious attention away from strong unconscious emotions that the mind does not want to experience.

Once I examined the effect of the repressed emotions in my life and understood the triggers or stressors that caused these repressed emotions to activate physical pain in my body, I began to realise that pain and addiction were one and the same thing, they had the same origin.

For alcoholics who are now drinking socially, it is beneficial to have an outlet to share experiences so that they can resolve new issues and bring them into the open, so they lose their power to create new pain or addiction.

This is the main function of the OTI recovery program and meetings, a place where like-minded people can socialize, reveal and heal their pain and enjoy a few drinks.

For the majority of people, who have very little repressed childhood experiences, they rarely if ever have the symptoms that are common for people who have them; e.g., migraine, chronic pain, irritable bowel syndrome, ulcers, addiction to alcohol, and addiction to illegal drugs or prescription drugs.

In the majority of cases, people who have had early childhood experiences and are able and given the opportunity to express them, never go on to develop these symptoms. However, where a nurturing or supportive environment in the home is not available, it is common for people to repress trauma and emotional issues.

In some instances, people who had normal childhoods and reached adolescence and adulthood without any major traumas, may not develop these symptoms until later in life when they experience stressors or major trauma that they are unable to handle, that they are unable to share or unable to express

This repression, even in later life, can result in addictive behaviours, physical pain and in some cases emotional pain like depression.

So for me and for many others who stopped drinking through Alcoholics Anonymous (AA) it became necessary for us, while in AA, to believe in a power greater than ourselves which AA called God, or a "God of your own understanding". This was Bill Wilson's greatest achievement. He developed the AA spiritual program. It worked, if you never wished to take a drink of alcohol again. It worked because it never became necessary to question whether one could drink or not.

In AA, it is necessary to fully accept that you can never drink safely again. To reinforce this you need to attend regular AA meetings.

The AA first step is acceptance that you are "powerless over alcohol" and so it became necessary to hand all your decisions to a higher power or a "God of your own understanding".

For me this is a rejection of personal responsibility for your own life. In Over the Influence (OTI) meetings, you accept that you are powerful over addiction and that your life is manageable by you.

AA at the time was necessary for me as I had no other knowledge about alcoholism. Like most people new to AA, I was suffering from extreme distress as a result of years of chronic alcoholism. So believing in a higher power or in God or in anything else that was asked of me was accepted without question. It saved my life. And because I knew no better and because I knew no other way or no other solution, I lived with this belief and this information for nearly 30 years of continuous sobriety in AA, and accepted that I could never drink again or it would be fatal.

This became so ingrained in my mind that to think about drinking again was frightening in itself. It was brainwashed into my life for nearly 30 years that this was a definite medical and scientific fact. But like all facts, if the source of the information that the fact is derived from is incorrect, then the fact is no longer true. It's just a belief that was held at the time when it was needed to help people recover from a fatal addiction. At the time there was no other way and no better knowledge.

I accepted all of the AA philosophy until I came to understand, acknowledge and accept the MindBody source of alcoholism and discovered its cure.

I now know, that thinking beyond this corrected fact, is really like curing my physical pain. Thinking beyond the old belief was not something that came naturally after the years of brainwashing that was necessary to keep me away from alcohol. However that brainwashing is no longer needed. The brain now knows what the cause of the addiction was and what the effect was and why it was 'needed' at the time.

The reason or function of addiction has been disclosed so it is no longer necessary and the brain needs to be told this. The brain now realises that I was a perfectly clear, fresh human being without any addiction, without any pain until the process of repression and diversion started, until my life of fear and anxiety started.

So a "God of my own understanding" was good for me for almost 30 years and God or a higher power of some sort is good for alcoholics when they need something to hang onto, to prevent them thinking of a reality where drink is okay.

But in my new reality, which is the truth for me, I know that taking a drink of alcohol is okay, and that acceptance of a higher power or a spiritual program is now a personal choice and not essential for everyone. I now have taken back personal responsibility for the rest of my new life.

With this new MindBody knowledge, it is irrelevant what your spiritual or religious leanings are, it is now up to the individual to cure themselves, and they can.

I now know that my life, my pain and my addiction are completely in my own control. I now know that I have power to heal all parts of my life; to heal my addiction permanently, to heal my pain permanently and to live without either of them.

This means, that with this knowledge and awareness, alcoholism and chronic pain are no longer an issue. Whether I drink or don't drink alcohol is not the issue because it's no longer an addiction.

My mind created the addiction to alcohol first, because it was the only thing at the time that completely prevented the repressed emotions from surfacing. It prevented them from surfacing in such a way that it was euphoric.

At times when alcohol was unable to create the diversion, suicide became another option to prevent the suppressed emotions from surfacing.

Once alcohol started to work it was like ecstasy, in that my life of not knowing who I was, of not knowing what was going on in my life, of not knowing what was going on in my mind, did not matter anymore once I had taken the drink.

This was the first stage of the addiction. Alcohol worked for a long while to hide those repressed emotions and to hide the new emotions that were being suppressed on a daily basis.

Alcohol itself then became the suppressor of the new alcoholic-created traumas in my life. It also became the manifestation of the old repressed emotions, just as physical pain did, later on in my life.

So the being that I am now, I have always been and it's only now that I realise this. The power of my being, the power of the 'I' of me is completely clear of addiction and of pain and always has been.

So when I live in the 'I' of me, when I'm living in my being and being who I am, addiction and pain do not exist or control my life. I can prevent future pain and addiction by acknowledging and exposing the stressors and triggers, the source and creators of pain and addiction in my life.

For me to suggest to a member of Alcoholics Anonymous that drinking socially is now possible, will be very frightening to them. The suggestion that it might be possible makes some people immediately nervous of me as if I was carrying some sort of disease. And I can fully understand that. I've been like that all my sober life. I was afraid to think any differently.

But now that I drink alcohol socially (after over 30 years of continuous sobriety in AA) and know where my addiction began and how it was manifested in physical, emotional and intellectual ways in my life, I know now that it is possible for anyone, previously addicted to alcohol, to drink socially again. I have exposed the purpose of addiction and my brain knows that I know this.

The departure from the tenets of AA felt very like the time I decided to leave a religious organization when I was a teenager and also like the time I left a secure job to set up my own business. It was a scary thing to do at the time. However I had a sense of excitement as I was leaving all of this behind and for the first time, truly being my own person. It felt like a huge load had been lifted from me.

In the religious organization I was secretly moved away from my colleagues before I left, in case they would catch the bug and leave too. But like then, I have to stand up and be counted and express my beliefs and be true to my new knowledge, awareness and experience.

There will be many who will feel threatened by this information, who will be afraid to follow my example, lest their lives get worse. There will be some who, to cement their reliance, commitment and dependence on AA, will say I was never an alcoholic in the first place.

For me, truth is life and life is truth and I have always put my head above the crowd when I believed in something, no matter what the consequences for myself.

I was unable to live with my physical pain and I was unable to live happily with my suppressed sober life and now I've cured both of them. It really does not matter whether I drink or don't drink anymore. I have a choice and have made the choice that drinking alcohol is not going to affect my life in any negative way and I have proven that it doesn't.

My mind made a decision when I took my first drink. It found that the effects of alcohol in me were the greatest diversion from the conscious eruption of my repressed, and ongoing suppressed emotions. The mind needed the diversion as a self-safety valve.

I have no need for this diversion anymore. I now know what was going on. I know what the source and creator of my addiction and physical pain was. The source has been exposed and has lost its power. MindBody awareness, knowledge and acceptance has cured them. I've come back to being who I am. I no longer need the escape or diversion that was provided by addiction and pain.

CHAPTER 13 The Physical Diversion

Like addiction, chronic pain is rampant throughout the Western world and statistics indicate that this epidemic is spreading. Many people suffer needlessly from pain diagnosed as migraines, tension headaches or chronic neck, back, abdominal and pelvic pain, when the real cause, like addiction, is MindBody related.

Millions of people, mostly women, suffer from the pain malady called Fibromyalgia, a disorder of the muscles that causes pain and tenderness all over the body.

After trying every known treatment, people are often told to just live with the pain, that there is no cure, and they are sometimes heavily medicated. Huge medical industries have arisen to treat these conditions, but the pain epidemic continues.

If you are suffering from chronic pain that appears to have no medical cause, the real cause, like the cause of addiction, may be MindBody related, what I will call from now on MindBody Pain or MBP.

To look at a typical scenario of someone with chronic pain; they have really bad pain, and they can't get rid of it. They go to a doctor and he or she tells them that they have a medical condition. The diagnosis might be back or neck pain presumably due to arthritis, a bulging disk or spinal stenosis. Or maybe the diagnosis was tension headache or migraine headache. Or maybe fibromyalgia or whiplash or chronic tendonitis, was the diagnosis. Or it might have been stomach pains or pelvic pains, with a diagnosis of irritable bowel syndrome or cystitis.

They were then prescribed medication. They took the medication and it didn't really help. Maybe they even had surgery, and that didn't help either. So they decided to explore alternative medicine. Maybe they took herbal remedies, vitamins or saw a chiropractor. And they might also have considered acupuncture, hypnosis, and even crystals, to heal the pain. But still the pain is there.

And they're not imagining or making up the pain. The pain is in their body and it's severe and very real.

The problem is the diagnosis! If their diagnosis is wrong, they can't get better. They may not have a serious disease. But they do have a medical condition. And they're not crazy. In fact, they're not any different from anybody else. The real problem is that their body is producing pain, because it's manifesting unresolved stress, possibly from as far back as their childhood, or from stressful events in their adulthood, or from stressful events in their present circumstances, and sometimes as a result of their personality traits. Their personality affects how they respond to stress and how much pressure they tend to put on themselves.

So, if this is your experience, then your mind has twisted your body into pain as a way to avoid some of the painful emotions that are inside you. If you haven't been helped by traditional or alternative medical care, your diagnosis may be MindBody related or a form of MindBody pain (MBP). And, most people have some form of MBP, I had! But you don't have to live the rest of your life with this pain. In fact, if you begin to understand this MindBody pain and recognize what causes it, you've taken a powerful first step, to healing your chronic pain, by reading this book.

With the information I am giving you, you may be able to get rid of the pain yourself, without drugs, without medical treatments (either conventional or alternative), and without counselling or psychotherapy. Results may occur immediately, or within three to four weeks, even though you may have been suffering for months or years. You don't have to go back and figure out all your unresolved emotional issues either, to cure this chronic pain. You might even become pain free (and addiction free) after reading this book.

You can break the connection between your mind and your physical pain (or addiction). You can start to use your mental energy to overcome your pain and rebuild your life. I know this is true, because I have done it myself. I've changed my understanding of the source of my pain. Now I can stop my body from producing MindBody pain that used to be created as a diversion for my repressed emotions and the stresses and strains of everyday life.

My experience of fully healing my own recurring chronic pain while waiting for surgery has motivated me to tell everyone how I did it. I Hope that what I tell you will help you or someone you know to overcome their chronic pain, if the cause of their pain has the same source as mine. I cured my chronic pain permanently and I never needed surgery or medication.

I had tried all the conventional treatments; doctors, back specialists, acupuncture, complementary/alternative therapy, chiropractors, medication, orthopaedic surgeons, rheumatologists and nothing worked for me. Nobody could heal the pain.

My severe physical pain continued and was seriously affecting my life. I had been diagnosed with a variety of bone and disc problems. In the end, surgery was the only option given to me. And I was on the verge of disc removal and bone fusion surgery when I found out about MBP and I cured myself completely!

The information I am giving you is backed up by 40 years of medical research by the top medical practitioners and neuroscientists around the world. However, it is still not part of mainstream medicine.

I would advise, that before taking any of this information on board, that you make sure you have a thorough medical check by a qualified Doctor and have completed all their required scans and tests. Make sure you have had enough testing to rule out a purely physical cause for your pain, or other symptoms.

If you are suffering from chronic pain and/or other symptoms, that your doctors have been unable to diagnose, treat, or cure, you may have MBP.

So, to start healing your chronic pain, I want you to consider that feelings generated in infancy and childhood, permanently reside in your unconscious and could be responsible for the psychological and physical symptoms you suffer from, throughout your life.

Strong painful, embarrassing and threatening feelings, like rage, grief and shame are repressed in our unconscious. These repressed emotions constantly strive to come to consciousness – that is, they want to escape from the unconscious and come into the open and consciously manifest in your life.

Our chronic pain (and addiction) is created to prevent these repressed feelings from becoming conscious, by diverting attention, from the realm of the emotions, to that of the physical, and causing pain in the body.

MBP often starts in childhood or adolescence, with many people first developing headaches, stomach aches, dizziness, fatigue, anxiety or other symptoms while they are still very young. And then later in life they start to develop chronic pain; whether it's in their back or their neck, their knee, or their stomach, or they have fibromyalgia, or irritable bowel syndrome, or other painful conditions.

Where do the repressed emotions (like hurt, shame, resentment, embarrassment, anger, guilt, humiliation, anxiety, fear or worry) come from?

The three main sources are; 1) from emotional distress in childhood. This could be related to emotional, physical or sexual abuse. Even if we have made peace with it, the distress is still there and is a potential source of unpleasant feelings, and 2) from everyday issues such as worry about work, about your children, about your parents, about relationships, about finances, and many more everyday situations and 3) our personalities also predispose us to these troubling emotions and cause stress, especially if we have high expectations and place great demands on ourselves, or if we are a perfectionist, or conscientious, and always going out of our way to help others, at our own expense.

So we have stresses and strains from daily life, we have the residue of anger from childhood and other internal conflicts and we have the stresses imposed by the personality. Keeping these emotions hidden often feels safer, feels much safer in fact, than ranting and raving like a lunatic in public. But they do try to escape and are instead expressed in the body, as severe physical pain.

I discovered that my repressed emotions, especially anger and rage, and my personality traits, were a major factor in bringing on my chronic pain, and as mentioned earlier, my addictive personality.

I tended to be a perfectionist, I was also compulsive, and I was highly conscientious and ambitious. I was driven, I was self critical, and I set very high standards for myself and was often successful.

And in parallel with these traits I had a compulsion to please and to be a good person, to be helpful and non-confrontational. And as a result of emotional abuse as a child, I had quite low self-esteem, no matter how many successes I had. And I always had a strong need to prove myself and to seek approval. I also had a strong drive to be helpful, often to the extent of sacrificing my own needs.

So unknowingly I created a lot of anger and other strong emotions in my life and I repressed them, because these strong emotions did not fit with the image of myself that I wanted the world to see. And most of the time I was not aware that these emotions were repressed or part of a bigger reservoir of rage, that I was carrying, and that I was continually filling up during my life.

In relation to chronic pain, your pain may be in the lower back, accompanied by numbness, tingling or weakness in any part of one or both legs. It might be in the neck or the shoulder with pain, numbness, tingling or weakness in one or both arms or hands. It could be in the elbow, the wrist, the fingers, the hip area, the knee, the ankle, the top or bottom of the foot.

It might be in the stomach or you might be getting continuous allergies from a rundown immune system. You might be getting recurring headaches or severe migraine. And sometimes you might be diagnosed with fibromyalgia, or diagnosed with a tear in a muscle or tendonitis. Or maybe you have all of the above, which keep moving around the body at different times.

Your pain may be worse during the day or at night. It may be severe when you wake up and try to get up, gradually improving during the day or it may be the opposite. It may be aggravated or improved by sitting, standing or walking. You may be afraid to bend or lift.

You may not be able to work or do any exercise. You may be afraid to do anything physical, no matter how easy the task or manoeuvre. You may be continually distressed and depressed because of the pain.

And maybe you have continued to be active despite the pain, working your way through it, despite the agony. You may get pain at strange illogical times. One of my own experiences was getting an ankle sprain when I was sitting on a bus, and I ended up on crutches.

Most of the time I was under the impression that something was wrong with my ankle, my back, my neck or my shoulder, that it was a structural defect like a deterioration or degeneration of parts of my spine, or a bulging or herniated disk.

My doctor supported this notion and his diagnosis was supported by X-rays and MRI scans. Little did I know at the time that eighty percent of people with a similar scan result have no physical pain. It's just normal wear and tear.

Since I cured my chronic pain through MindBody awareness, my back still has these same abnormalities (or wear and tear, to give them their proper name), but I have no pain!

At the time my life was dominated by pain and it moved around to different parts of my body. And as I mentioned, I tried all the regular treatments including medication, and then I was getting ready for surgery. I was continually warned to be careful, not to make it worse, and was limited in my ability to move around. Pressure tests on the long tendons on the side of both my thighs, and on my back and shoulders revealed lots of tenderness and pain.

I now know that the structural abnormalities identified in the scans were not the cause of the pain I had. The pain, the stiffness, the burning, the pressure, the numbness, the tingling and weakness, were all caused by mild oxygen deprivation in the muscles, nerves and tendons, in the locations of the pain.

Although the pain was severe, I discovered that it was harmless and could be reversed without any residual damage.

My brain had seen fit to reduce the blood flow to these areas, causing the distressing symptoms. Why, you might ask. Well, the severe pain, caused by the reduced blood flow, was a diversion mechanism, preventing my repressed rage and other powerful emotions, escaping from my unconscious, and stopping them coming into my consciousness. It was a self-safety valve, causing pain as a distraction to prevent these intolerable feelings and rage from surfacing.

When I realized this, I suddenly became aware of the many different repressed psychological factors in my own life, that were responsible for my pain, and that were being triggered by the stresses of my daily life. My unconscious pot of rage had boiled over and wanted conscious attention, but the brains self-safety valve instead diverted my attention to the body, by creating severe physical pain and many other symptoms. For some people these symptoms could include depression and addiction.

So, if you have chronic pain that is not responding to traditional or complementary medicine, to start the healing process, the first thing you need to do, is to reject the structural diagnosis and accept that you are more than a mechanical body, that your MindBody interaction may be the cause of your pain – not just the body!

When the pain was in my back, the pain did not stop until I was able to say to myself; "I have a normal back, I now know that the pain is due, to a basically harmless condition, initiated by the brain to serve a psychological purpose, that is, to get me to focus on my body and not on the rage and other strong emotions, that I have repressed in my unconscious".

I began to realize that the resolution to my pain would come from understanding and knowledge, and not from any structural intervention. So, to cure the pain, I first had to reject the "physical only" reason for the severe pain. I had to acknowledge the psychological basis for the pain.

As I mentioned earlier, it has been proven that a lot of the structural abnormalities found on X rays and MRI scans, are normal changes associated with activity and aging, and most of us have these, without any pain. So, in my case I had to dismiss the structural diagnosis as faulty, as it did not accurately explain the pain location or the fact that the pain moved around to different parts of my body.

Also the pain often occurred at the wrong time; for example when I was resting comfortably in bed. I have also known many people since then, who were block laying or doing some other heavy physical activity all day, and who only got pain in the morning whenever they were heading into a stressful work situation.

Thousands of people with a large variety of structural changes in their spine or were diagnosed with fibromyalgia for instance, have since recovered completely in days or weeks after learning about what was going on in their MindBody interaction.

Structural abnormalities are widespread and are seldom the cause of chronic pain. In 1994, a US medical research team reported, that in a group of 98 men and women diagnosed by MRI scans, 64 had herniated disks, disc bulges and protrusions, and none of these 64 ever had back pain!

So, just to say it again, the structural abnormalities are not always the cause of pain, as in my case. And as I discussed earlier, alcohol is not the cause of alcoholism, or drugs the cause of drug addiction. Like addiction, chronic pain, is often a MindBody creation.

Some people with a herniated disk shown on CT scan or MRI have back and leg pain in roughly the right location to explain their symptoms. However when they recover completely through awareness MBP we know for definite, that the herniated disc was never the problem.

The mind is ingenious, when it wishes to create a physical distraction. The mind is aware of everything that goes on in the body. There's a famous book called the "Molecules of Emotion" by Prof Candace Pert, a molecular scientist. And from her work you can clearly see, that the body and mind are continually interacting and communicating, and know each other intimately.

The mind knows the site of herniated discs, of meniscus tears in knee joints; it knows the site of tears of the rotator cuff at the shoulder. My experience has shown that the brain will often initiate pain where a structural abnormality already exists! It is one of the best ways to keep your attention focused on the body.

The mind will also induce pain at the site of an old injury; in my case, my old knee injury and my old ankle injury – yet awareness and acceptance of its MindBody creation stopped the pain instantly and I was able to resume normal physical activities.

In the case of my ankle, I was unable to walk and was on crutches. I had forgotten what was going on in my life emotionally, but as soon as I remembered the MBP cure process, I stopped the pain instantly, and in a few days I was back playing tennis again.

A few years ago I had a severe attack on my neck and was wearing a neck brace during the day and sleeping with an orthopaedic pillow at night. I was in agony. I couldn't turn my head and was also receiving physiotherapy. Again, I fixed this myself instantly once I remembered that it was MBP related.

Another time I was suffering from an ulcer. I was put on ulcer medication. And again, I fixed this myself instantly with the MBP awareness.

But sometimes, like myself, you will forget what's going on in your life at the time, that is, the trigger for the pain, and you may start to go down the standard medical route, before realizing that you have the cure yourself, if it is MindBody related.

In all of these occasions of pain, my brain was desperately trying to divert attention from rage and other strong emotions, in my unconscious, by using the physical pain. On each occasion, after I recognized it for what it was I was able to pinpoint what the emotions were that triggered the pain that had again overloaded the unconscious reservoir, which had been filling since I was a child.

The brain's attempt to divert attention to the body, rather than to the repressed rage, is an automatic reaction of the mind. It is not based on logic or reason, but done just as a self protective method, to prevent you experiencing the intolerable repressed emotions, many of which we have no idea what they are or when they were repressed.

To stop this automatic system we have to bring reason to the process, that is, we have to bring our conscious mind into action. So we can and I did, influence the unconscious automatic reactions, first by this MBP knowledge and then by the application of a conscious thought process.

This is not a theory – it worked for me 100% and has worked for thousands more. I am completely pain free today. There are Doctors all over the world who have been doing this MindBody work for over 40 years.

So just a quick recap. The threat of the painful emotions exploding into your consciousness must be of sufficient strength, to necessitate the production of severe physical pain or the creation of addiction or depression.

The mind fears that the unconscious rage or other strong emotions that you have repressed, will break out into consciousness, destroying our image of ourselves in front of others, so it focuses our attention on the body, by creating pain, ranging from minor pains, like stress in your shoulder, to severe chronic pain, in many parts of your body.

And for some people, as I mentioned earlier, it creates addiction and depression as the diversion mechanism.

The reasons for your repressed rage, and the other strong emotions that you carry inside could be trauma in your infancy and childhood. And this can occur in any family. It doesn't have to be a dysfunctional family. Your personality traits are another reason for repression, for example if you have low self esteem, if you are a perfectionist, if you are a hostile or aggressive type of person, if you carry a lot of guilt or shame, if you are a people pleaser, or if you are over-dependant on others.

Also, stressful events like the death of a spouse, divorce, personal injury or illness, relationship difficulties, work issues, retirement, finances, business difficulties or moving house can cause anger, rage, and repression of emotions.

Other reasons for the creation and repression of anger and rage are that our basic needs are not being met, for example, our need to excel, to achieve, and to succeed, to be liked and then being self-critical and sensitive to criticism.

As I mentioned earlier, my addiction and chronic pain was a direct result of anger and rage that was repressed in my unconscious. As well as this, my consciously suppressed anger kept adding to this reservoir of repressed rage in the unconscious.

The anger that is known to us plays a role in the creation of pain when it is suppressed, that is the anger that we know about; but it is not nearly as important as the anger that is generated in the unconscious as a result of childhood experiences, internal conflicts and the stresses and strains of daily life.

The first time I had an attack of chronic pain in my life was a number of years ago. And it was triggered by a conscious event in my life that made me extremely angry at the time. As I could not, or was afraid to act on the anger consciously, it was suppressed and it unleashed severe pain in my body.

I realise now, that my unconscious reservoir of repressed pain, had reached its limit and could not keep the lid on any longer, and the emotional trigger at that time, (which was the conscious anger that I was suppressing), caused the unconscious to manifest the pain in my body.

The resulting physical pain lasted for a long time, until I discovered the MBP link and then I fixed the pain myself. Over the years this happened again and again when emotional stressors or triggers were present, the pain appearing in different locations in my body each time.

However, sometimes, knowing that unconscious feelings are the cause of the chronic pain is not enough to get rid of it. We must seek to fully recognize the reasons for the rage to fully understand the process.

Bad experiences in infancy and childhood make the earliest contributions to our reservoir of anger and rage, plus the personality traits that I mentioned earlier, like, low self-esteem, perfectionism, guilt, and dependency. Even happy events like getting married or going on holidays can trigger these dormant feelings and create physical pain.

Remember, it's an illogical process, so don't use logic to try and understand it – just accept it and see what happens.

Put too much water in a saucepan and it will spill out, if you heat it up with the lid on it will explode into steam. Compare the steam to the reduction in blood flow to your nerves, muscle and tendons.

Instead of holding the undesirable emotions and rage in, the unconscious mind deoxygenates parts of the body.

So whenever you are aware of the pain, you must consciously think of the repressed rage and the reasons for it. This will contradict what the brain is trying to do, that is, getting you to focus on the body and it will undo the brain's strategy.

So focus on those unpleasant, threatening thoughts and feelings and deny the pain its purpose, which is to divert your attention from those feelings, to the body.

When the pain is severe, it's difficult to concentrate on feelings, but you must regard the process as a contest in which your conscious will is pitted against the unconscious.

So to heal your pain you need to talk to your brain. This might sound silly but it works. It worked for me and thousands more.

So when you understand the MBP cure, say with conviction to your brain "I know what you are up to"! In this way, your conscious mind addresses the unconscious and the more forcefully you do it the better.

So after you accept this cure and it works for you, when you feel the next twinge of pain, which often is the first sign of a severe bout coming on, let your unconscious know that you know what it is at and then, as in my case the pain will disappear.

So tell your mind that you know what it is doing, that you know that the physical pain is harmless. It is severe and may be disabling, but it is harmless.

You will be able to resume all your physical activities once you cure the pain. The physical pain is just a distraction from the repressed rage, so tell your mind that you no longer intend to be diverted or intimidated.

In most cases it doesn't matter whether you know what the rage is about, to cure the pain – you only need the knowledge, the 'why' and 'how' it is created. You can even tell your mind to increase the blood flow to the muscles, tissues, nerves and tendons that are involved, but this is not necessary. The brain is in constant communication with the rest of your body, so tell it what you know.

If you are suffering from pain at the moment, it is a good idea to first write down all the stresses and pressures in your life, since they all contribute to your inner rage.

We all have self imposed pressures especially if we are perfectionist or trying to please everyone. And of course we all have everyday pressures – whether we are single, married, working, unemployed, on holidays, have children, whatever. A biggie for a lot of people is the anger left over from childhood, and especially if you suffered emotional, sexual or physical abuse.

When you make your stressor list, you might be shocked to see the list you come up with – I was and it went back to my infancy and childhood.

You might think it will make things worse if you look at all the troubles in your life. In fact it is the opposite. When you look at your stressors in the light of this new MBP knowledge, it will cure your pain.

It is our failure to realize the impact of these emotions on the inner mind that leads to the pain. By identifying and dealing with our sources of pressure and anger, we reduce their negative impact in the unconscious. As I have said all along, the purpose of the pain and other symptoms is to keep your attention focused on the body.

However, when you go through the MBP process and the pain disappears, if you are still fearful of physical activity or of injury to any part of your body, your battle has not been completely won.

The pain will return unless you overcome those fears. So for me I resumed normal physical activity once the pain was gone, when I had fully convinced myself of the cure.

After I healed my ankle pain, I waited a few weeks before playing tennis again. Unfortunately when you have been constantly exposed and bombarded with information, on the so-called fragility of the human body, especially the back, it might take you months to become fully active again.

When I was in pain, I was told never to do this or that, do it this way; be careful, you'll hurt yourself. your spine is out of line, the discs are degenerated and the spinal bones are rubbing together, one of your legs is shorter than the other, people weren't meant to walk upright, you've got flat feet, don't swim the crawl or the breast stroke, don't arch your back, never sleep on your stomach, always bend your knees when you bend at the waist, don't lift, don't do sit-ups and on and on and on. All of these warnings kept my attention riveted on my body, which as I have mentioned earlier, is the brain's intention.

After I cured myself, my path to resumption of full physical activity, without fear, sometimes was immediate, sometimes it was slow, but it was always steady and progressive. I had mild pain at the beginning, until the full cure became apparent and was reinforced by my physical activity. The brain took its time to change its programming. So take your time, try and try again – you will prevail in the end – I did and thousands of others have as well.

Don't start physical activity too soon, as the brain and body have to agree, and the brain's reprogramming may not be as fast as the body's. The brain needs to accept your move to physical activity. I accepted the MBP knowledge and it worked, and has worked every time. As I said, I am pain free and play tennis and cycle every week.

After you accept the MBP knowledge, it may be better to wait until the pain diminishes completely and your confidence is strong and the brain is on board and reprogrammed.

The goal of the MBP knowledge is to change the unconscious mind's reaction to emotional states. When this has been accomplished, pain will cease.

This is not just a cure, but prevention of future pain, as you will 'remember' what to do if it happens again, as it did to me many times.

Unfortunately I stayed in excruciating pain a few times, until I 'remembered' the MBP cure.

So remember, you are not treating pain anymore, you are treating the cause of pain which gives you a permanent cure! You are using knowledge, of the cause, to cure the pain, which is the effect created by the repressed emotions.

In some cases, like my back, and neck and my ulcer, the cessation of pain was instant, but in others it took a bit more time until the fear of physical activity went.

I cannot say this often enough; the purpose of the pain is to divert attention from what is going on emotionally and to keep you focused on the body. It is a contest for conscious attention.

For the majority of people, to heal their pain, you do not need to experience the emotions or bring them to consciousness. In my case all I needed to do was know that it was repressed rage that was causing my pain, and the pain disappeared as soon as I 'knew' this fact and accepted it.

So reflect on the repressed rage and think about all the pressures that produced it from childhood to the present day. It could be something current that is enraging you and triggering, your reservoir of rage.

I discovered that all of my physical pain, and it was severe pain, was of psychological rather than structural origin, and its role was to divert attention from frightening feelings. The pain was physical and severe, but its origin was psychological.

Most people get better simply by shifting their attention from the physical to the psychological – some others need more information and assistance.

In every case, MBP knowledge is essential to the cure, for by making yourself aware of what is going on, both physically and psychologically, you frustrate the brain's strategy.

By changing the focus of attention from the body to the mind we render the pain useless, we take away its purpose, and reveal what it is trying to hide. It may be necessary for some people to experience the emotions, like rage or profound sadness, before the pain will cease – but in the majority of cases this is not necessary.

You may be aware of the pain, the anger, the sadness in your life, but until you accept and acknowledge them as the source of your physical pain, the pain will persist.

Knowledge of the emotions is not enough in itself; you must accept that they are the cause of your physical pain, before the pain will go away.

This cure only works when you decide to look at it seriously. You have to make a strong effort to apply it. You must either believe that it can work for you, or you must be so desperate that you will try very hard to do it, even if you don't believe it.

By nature I'm very sceptical. I didn't believe that my mind could solve my physical pain. However I was desperate. I had tried everything else to cure the pain and I was still in constant pain. So I had nothing to lose but try it and my pain was cured 1one hundred percent by this MBS knowledge alone!

So, first make a commitment to relook at your pain from another angle. You have nothing to lose, but your pain. Concentrate, and see if the personality types, the repressed anger and your current life stressors apply to you. Look for similarities not differences.

When you write down your list of stressors, check every day to see what problems might be bothering you, what might be in your life and in your mind that is causing you pain? Think about the areas I mentioned;

like work or school pressure, or relationships or responsibilities, or financial matters, or whatever else is going on.

Be as specific as possible, when you're writing down your list. No use saying "I'm worried about work". You have to list the 'whys'. Try to indentify every possible item you can think of. Pay attention to all areas of your life, big and small stressors. The conscious suppressed big ones can cause pain in themselves, and both big and small stressors can trigger the old repressed ones.

Go beyond the obvious ones, and think about what might be hidden in your life. Consider real and imagined fears that might be troubling you.

Once you have identified your problems, divide them into two categories; those that you can do something about, and those that are beyond your control, and be realistic about where each one fits. The ones you can do something about, start taking action on them. Do whatever you can to correct them, or try to at least.

The ones that you have no control over tell yourself, that you know they bother you, but you must accept them – and more important, you are not going to let them cause you any more pain. Tell your mind this, strongly! It works!

Remember, you don't have to eliminate your problems for this to cure to work. You just have to be aware and accept the MBP process.

Think about what you are like – what is it in you that lets these problems create such pain – again I mentioned some of these earlier; are you a perfectionist, are you easily angered, are you highly motivated, a high achiever, are you compulsive or impatient, do you have childhood issues, are you helping everyone at your own expense.

Those were some parts of my personality that led my mind to develop pain. It started in my back and then moved everywhere else; to my knee, my neck, my shoulder, my head, my ankle, my stomach, etc. However, you don't need to be like me in any way to develop the pain. Try to learn what is inside of you that needs the distraction.

What permits the pain to develop in the first place, and to persist? Be honest with yourself! What are you avoiding looking at? You don't have to change your personality for the cure to work – you just have to understand the cause, which I have already outlined.

Whenever you have any issues in the future that angers or bothers you, say to yourself : "Okay I don't like that, but I'm not going to let it go to my back, or my head, or my neck and cause me pain". This is prevention as well as cure.

Easy does it, but do it! Take small steps at first. Look for tiny improvements. Find something you can do that doesn't hurt quite as much as it used to. Go slowly, and you'll notice over time that your pain will recede and the pain in your body will improve. Build on the small steps and the slightest improvement will keep you on track and will encourage you.

So when you feel pain in the future, ask yourself; "What's going on in my life or in my mind to make this hurt". Take a close look internally, and see what's going on for you emotionally at that time. What is causing your pain to flare up? What is going on in your life to trigger your repressed emotions?

Pain is depressing and discouraging. So don't give up! There is hope and I have cured all of my pain one hundred percent. But you must put in the time and effort for it to work. This is not traditional, complementary or alternative medicine. It is MindBody medicine.

This is not a placebo effect. This is not based on blind faith; it is based on finding and accepting the cause of pain. Placebos are temporary fixes, this is not. Many standard treatments have a placebo effect – including surgery, where patients develop pain in other areas of their body after surgery. The brain simply moves the pain to another location or another organ of the body, so that the distraction can continue.

Some people have had successful back surgery, only to develop ulcer problems afterwards, and when that was brought under control by medication, they developed severe neck pain, and on and on – as happened in my own case.

Often pain will recur at the site of an old injury. The mind is very smart, as I mentioned already. This cure is a process of education; - again, blind faith is not involved. You must conclude that what I say is logical and reasonable, satisfying yourself that the pain is a MindBody related issue. The cure is almost always permanent.

Like me, many people have tried every known treatment for their pain. Some have had surgery and their focus was kept on structural issues, and their fear deepened and the pain persisted.

With this cure, when you find the true reason for your pain and realize that you have a normal body, you then enlist the power of your mind to heal the body and it WORKS! You will be cured by learning to be aware of the nature of this MindBody interaction.

You may have to hear this repeatedly before it sinks in. I did! If pain persists despite this knowledge I would advise you to look deeper at the issues in your life. Usually you are not aware that you have anger and rage because it is unconscious. Being made aware of the existence of unconscious rage, and the reasons for it, is one of the primary therapeutic ingredients.

Pain in itself can make you feel enraged in a never ending vicious cycle – never knowing when the next attack will come or how severe it will be.

Being partially restricted in physical activities and finding it difficult to make plans, is also very enraging. When you learn that you can take control and rid yourself of this terrible scourge, it is exhilarating!! You will feel empowered to do many things that you thought were previously impossible!

As I mentioned earlier, rage often has its source in childhood trauma, and it may be as simple as feeling left out in a large family. It doesn't have to be physical, sexual or emotional abuse. And remember you do not have to remove any of the stressors in your life to cure the pain – you just need to acknowledge that they are what is causing it, and the pain disappears.

The rage is repressed, we often do not feel it, and therefore we cannot undo it, but we can undo its affects in the body!

You don't need to change your personality or stop trying to be perfect or good. We remain basically the same person we've always been, but our pain goes. Even if you go to emotional depths with a psychoanalyst, your personality is not going to change that much. However, the better we know ourselves, the less the feelings of rage will frighten us. It's acknowledging the cause that is the cure.

Throughout our lives we will continue to generate some anger and rage, but we can stop it causing physical pain, by just using our mind.

So again, knowledge, not change, produces the cure. Pain symptoms, like mine that were present for years, may stop in days or weeks, using your new knowledge and the power of your mind. Understanding and accepting the nature of MindBody pain is an intellectual process, it's a function of the conscious mind.

As the MindBody pain originates in the unconscious, these new ideas must penetrate and be accepted there, for the pain to cease. However, if the emotions are frightening enough, the mind will not let go easily, and may hold tightly to its distraction strategy, fearing that these emotions might become conscious. The mind decides it cannot do without the pain, and it will fight hard to keep it that way. So you may have to be very persistent.

The majority of people do not need psychotherapy or counselling. However, if the MindBody pain is not going away easily, then psychotherapy may be useful.

A trained psychotherapist can explore the unconscious and make you aware of the frightening, embarrassing or unacceptable feelings that are hidden there. However this will only help to cure the pain if the psychotherapist understands and accepts the MBP process, its cause and its effect.

As I said earlier, knowledge of the repressed emotions, especially rage and their MBP effect, is usually enough to cure your pain. The majority of people do not need to go any deeper, and do not require counselling or psychotherapy. You can heal your own pain with this MBP knowledge - I Did!

Sometimes your pain moves around. Your pain can move around to different locations, involving different muscles, nerves and tendons. It can also manifest in different symptoms.

However, like myself, when the pain returned in a different location a year later, locking my neck in severe pain (which was related to stressors in my life at the time), I had forgotten the MBP cure and started working with physiotherapists, taking pain killers, using special cushions etc - until one day I 'remembered' what was going on and more importantly why it was going on, and after talking to my brain I healed the pain instantly.

I did the same 'forgetting' with an ulcer and also pains in other locations, including migraine. Remembering the MBP knowledge, I was able to heal them all permanently.

Knowledge will fix it every time, when you tell your brain that you know what it is doing! And in the future, you will have rapid disappearance of new pain as soon as you realize what's going on.

The pain is due to mild oxygen deprivation, and the autonomic nervous system can change the rate of blood flow in seconds if it chooses, so you have control. Talk to your brain and the pain goes away. It's hard to believe, but it's very true and it works!

Pain and emotional turmoil are creations of the brain for the purpose of avoidance, and can substitute for each other at times.

So it may be physical or emotional pain that you experience – or both. So for example, you may have depression, addiction or physical pain as the avoidance mechanism or you may have all of them. With MBS knowledge you can cure both them all.

Acknowledgement and acceptance of the idea is essential to recovery. We are much stronger than we know, and we have the capacity to influence what is going on in our bodies. But we must get the MBP knowledge, understand it, accept it, and put it to use, by letting our brain know, that we know, what it is up to.

The pain symptoms are essentially harmless, though the severity of your pain may make that hard to believe at times. There is no permanent physical damage done. You can reverse the situation, and have no pain or any other after effects.

Knowledge of the MBS process and most particularly knowledge of its emotional source, is essential and results in the cure. Our greatest enemies are fear and misinformation.

Do not judge the unconscious mind by the accepted rules of logic and rationality that are characteristic of the conscious mind.

So, what does 'cured' mean, for me? For me, "cured" meant that my chronic pain and addiction went completely.

In relation to chronic pain, sometimes it went instantly; sometimes it took a day or two. And I'm talking about severe disabling pain and I have no pain today. "Cured" also meant that I was ready to engage in unrestricted physical activity, and now play tennis and cycle every day. I have no fear of any kind of physical activity, and I stopped all forms of physical and medical treatment. Cured also meant that I was able to take an alcoholic drink socially without any of the addictive compulsion setting in.

All of the above had to be present to prove to my brain that I knew what it was doing, that I was no longer misled by its MBP distraction, and that I was no longer intimidated by it or afraid. My logical conscious mind had unmasked my illogical unconscious mind.

Physiotherapists do an excellent job, but if your pain is due to MBP, that is, it is MBP related, physiotherapy will keep you thinking physically and not psychologically.

Fortunately, many Physiotherapists are now aware of MBP and its cure, and integrate it into their own work. So when you cure the pain, you can discontinue the exercises designed to protect the back, as they keep your mind focused on a structural problem, which you don't have!

Obviously, it's important to keep reasonably fit, and remember that physical exercise of any sort is good for your mind and your body and always warm up before any strenuous athletic exercises.

Remember that your pain will continue if you have not established and accepted the connection between the physical and psychological. So no matter what you do, whether its medication or therapy, if you fail to acknowledge that your pain is caused by a harmless circulatory alteration induced by the brain, your pain will continue.

The unconscious reservoir of rage and other unacceptable emotions reduces blood flow to your nerves, muscles, tendons and tissues, deoxygenating them, causing pain all over the body, moving around to different locations.

The anger you know about and express is not the anger causing your pain. MBP is a response to anger or rage and other emotions that are generated in the unconscious (in which case you are not aware of them most of the time). MBP can also be a response to conscious anger that you are suppressing.

MBP is not a response to conscious anger that you feel or express! And this is a very important distinction.

Psychologists interested in such conditions as fibromyalgia and chronic pain, focus on what they see, that is, the perceived emotions like anxiety, depression and hostility, for example. However I consider these disorders to also be outward manifestations of MBP, so it's not just physical pain that is used as a distraction by the mind!

Keep in mind that we repress anger that violates our image of ourselves. For example, if you have a strong need to seek approval from everyone, and someone does something that angers you, you will automatically repress that anger, because it destroys your image of yourself as a nice guy or nice girl. We get angry inside and do not allow it out.

Anger that you are aware of may be displaced anger. For example, you become very angry at something unimportant, like traffic jams or poor service in a restaurant, and you express it this way instead of expressing it to your spouse or parent, because to do it to them is not allowed by your mind.

Often the personality traits that make you calm are stimulating a great deal of rage internally. Sometimes the child in you is often saying "I want to be taken care of and you are taking care of everyone else instead". This causes internal conflict that is repressed and hidden, causing anger and rage in the unconscious.

Great copers tend to put great pressure on themselves by not sharing with others, and the self doesn't like this. People often don't know HOW angry they are, or how much anger they have inside, or that their anger is responsible for their physical pain.

Remember, there's nothing seriously wrong with you if you have MBP. MBP symptoms are universal in Western society. They don't imply any mental or emotional illness or abnormality of any kind. Everyone that I've ever met has MBP to some degree or another, at some time in their lives, and we all have it at different levels of severity.

As an example of minor everyday physical reactions to emotional events; when we are embarrassed our face turns red, when we are asked to speak in front of 1,000's of people, sometimes our stomach will tighten up, when we have a stressful day, we may get a headache or a knot in our shoulder.

Almost everyone I have ever met has some physical symptoms due to stress and their reactions to it. With chronic pain, the severity of your pain, relates directly to the strength and size of your reservoir of repressed emotions. Temporary fixes will only move the pain to new locations and will continue to do so until you find and accept this MBP knowledge and cure the pain yourself permanently!

To recap, MBP occurs when the stresses of life trigger repressed emotions in our unconscious that cause our bodies to react by producing physical and sometimes emotional symptoms.

The symptoms, such as pain, are real. They are very real. They are not imagined or "in your head." The most important things for you to realize, is that your emotions are very powerful forces, that can cause physical symptoms, also psychological symptoms and finally, that if you have a form of Mind Body Pain you are not crazy. I know this because I'm not crazy and I have had MBP.

Your pain, addiction and depression can be triggered by current or past stressors, by worry, by anxiety, by fear, by anger and by many other emotions that come with being human.

It often depends on how full your reservoir of rage is at the time, as to how much everyday stressors you can suppress, without getting severe pain. When these current stressors overload the repressed reservoir, you will have continuous pain and misery until you get and accept the MBP knowledge.

CHAPTER 14 Basic meditation Tools

If your addiction and chronic pain is MindBody Pain (MBP) related, you can heal yourself NOW with the knowledge and information I have just given you. You don't need to do anything or listen to anything else.

Read this book as often as you like. Repetition is important. Some people have a 'lightbulb moment' on their first reading and cure themselves instantly. Others cure themselves after a few readings or after going to Over The Influence (OTI) meetings.

Remember, you have to think your way out of MindBody pain and this is often easier to do in solitude and quietness.

To stop your racing mind, or your 'monkey mind' as it's often called, Mindfulness Meditation (MM) can be very useful. Set a time each day and think about what it takes to get better and mindfully meditate on the stressors in your life. This will remove their impact, stopping them creating physical pain and other symptoms.

Mindfulness Meditation (MM) is a great way to investigate how your inner turmoil is playing out physically, and causing the pain. It is a great practice to do every morning, but you can take regular short MM breaks during the day as well, whether you are at home or at work.

Stressful situations come and go in everyone's life, but you can deal with them through MM, by recognizing these emotions for what they are, and not allowing them to be held inside, and not allowing them to cause physical or psychological symptoms in your life.

You can bring MM to every part of your life; when you're walking, eating, washing the dishes, driving, whatever and it will calm you down and relieve stress.

Rethinking and re-creating stressful situations in your head leads to increased stress and leads to resentment, to anger and to rage.

MM helps to create space between the stressors and your responses to them, and to ask yourself each time "Is this useful?" when there's something stressful going on in your head.

MM has been compared to a software upgrade for the brain, and has been proven by Neuroscientists studying long-term meditators under MRI scanners, that it improves your life by making permanent changes to your brain structure. It stops your 'monkey mind' from jumping all over the place and making wrong reactive decisions in your life.

MM will make you aware of what is happening right Now and neutralizes the voice in your head that is full of judgments, desires, assumptions and crazy plans. And, you'll tend to have less emotional hangovers and learn to respond and not to react.

As an added bonus, MM will also increase your creativity, your leadership abilities, and make you more focused. So, create a new body with exercise and create a new mind with Mindfulness Meditation (MM).

The well known and popular meditations I have introduced below are taken from many types of belief systems. To make them easier to use, read them out and record them for yourself. Most smartphones now a have a recording device and having the recordings on your phone means that these Mindfulness meditations will be available to you at all times.

You can include your own beliefs in the meditations if you wish, to make them more personal and meaningful for you. However, you do not need to believe in God or any higher power for these to add powerful physical and emotional benefits to your life.

These meditation exercises will change and enhance your brain and make it grow for your benefit.

We are always in the presence of an infinite and eternal energy from which all things proceed. It can be called the 'I' of you, God or whatever is equivalent to God in your belief system.

So start to align your thoughts with the 'I' of you, so that you can be the creator of your own life. Your thoughts are expressed in words, so keep your thoughts and words positive at all times.

Your personality is made up of countless individual characteristics, peculiarities, habits, and traits of character. These are the result of your former method of thinking, but they have nothing to do with the real you. The real nature of your "I" is energy, and is the source of real power when you come into a realization of your true nature.

You must accept that the "I" of you is pain free and can also always drink safely.

Use Mindfulness Meditation on a daily basis, to quiet the senses, to seek inspiration, and to focus your mental activity on now.

Dwell in the consciousness of your unity with all things, the formless substance that permeates everything.

Hand your will and your life into the care and direction of this formless 'I', this energy, every day and accept that without this connection you cannot create, you can only compete.

Connection to this creative formless substance which permeates all things, is facilitated by gratitude for what you already have and gratitude for what you are about to create and receive.

This book is not allied with any sect, spiritual or religious organization. But, if you have a spiritual or religious leaning, then start each day by reading the 'Just for Today' prayer at the end of the book, and then hand your will and your life into the care and direction of your God using the 'Handing Over', prayer.

You can add in the other prayers; 'Prayer of St Francis' and 'Clearing Prayer' as you wish.

To complement your spiritual and religious leanings and further enhance your life, practice the remaining meditations which will change you physically as well as energetically.

The neural circuitry in your brain actually changes, when you practice Mindfulness Meditation on a daily basis.

Remember you don't have to believe in anyone or anything outside yourself to cure your pain or addiction. All you need is knowledge and acceptance of the source of your addiction. You have the cure within you. It doesn't matter whether you are an agnostic or atheist, or engage in spiritual or religious practices.

The following meditations will calm your thoughts and prepare you for deeper relaxation exercises. They will slow your body and mind down while concentrating on your breathing. Your thoughts will become fewer and your body will start to relax.

As you meditate, continually focus in the now and tell your thoughts to stop when they start to appear.

The meditations are taken from many different practices and have been used all over the world. They will improve your physical, emotional and cognitive health, adding years of greater happiness to your life. If you add these to your daily repertoire of activities, you will find that they have a very powerful effect on your life. They will boost your immune system, enrich your life at work, rest and play, and improve your relationships.

To achieve the greatest effect, combine as many of the meditation techniques as you feel comfortable with.

It is not easy to keep these MM practices up so persevere until it gets easier and they become a habit.

Remember that even if you led a dysfunctional addicted life up to now, your brain accepted it as okay, and it has allowed you to survive, no matter what the cost. It is not easy to change habits and it takes time to grow new connections that have been firmly set up over years.

Any disruption to the old circuits that allowed you to live with your addiction, pain and dysfunction, causes anxiety in the brain, but this is temporary, so keep meditating, make it a habit and grow a new life, physically, mentally and spiritually.

Commit to a few minutes meditation every day and then gradually build it up. It might be helpful to complete a meditation at the start of your OTI group meeting. It is often easier to be motivated when you have a few other people involved. In an OTI meeting you will be socializing with like-minded people.

Neuroscience has proven the benefits of meditation and has shown the physical changes that take place in the brain during meditation. These changes become permanent with practice and time. The more time you spend the greater the results.

If you are not going to an OTI meeting every day, then set a specific time each day to meditate, maybe first thing in the morning when you wake up, or after work, and maybe last thing at night.

You can stand, sit on a cushion, lie back in your favourite chair or lie down. Feel comfortable but don't doze off, so lying down at night might not work, unless you want to fall asleep. The more you meditate, the quicker your brain gets you into the desired state. If you wish, play sounds or music that has meaning for you.

Research suggests that meditation consistently takes the practitioner into deep states of consciousness. When compared to everyday awareness, the brain, during meditation, is operating in an unusual way. And, since the underlying mechanics of Mindfulness Meditation are theologically neutral, it can be integrated with any religious doctrine or creed and will be a great support in your new pain free and non-addicted life.

Meditation 1 Mind Relaxing the Body

In this first meditation I will introduce you to some basic breathing techniques, which you can use at any time, and you can also bring them into other meditations if you wish.

The Sanskrit word for breath is PRANA which means life force or vital energy. By regulating your breath you help to balance your energy field and help to shift blocked emotions that are causing pain throughout your body.

Research has continually shown that breathing exercises lower stress and anxiety, improve coping skills, improve your general sense of well-being, and improves self-esteem.

Conscious breathing can also integrate and eliminate negative energies that affect your mind and body.

Slow focused breathing triggers the body's relaxation response. It also increases dopamine levels in different parts of the brain during the first 10 minutes of meditation, which explains why the experience can be very pleasurable.

Deep breathing helps to calm your mind, so if you have trouble turning down your thoughts, deepen your breathing as you meditate.

So when you meditate, it is recommended that you start by breathing through your nose, because it turns out that nasal breathing increases the release of nitric oxide in your body and this improves the functioning of your lungs and your circulatory system. Deep breathing also helps to keep the internal temperature of your brain in balance.

So our first meditation practice begins with a breathing exercise, the most basic meditation practice in the world.

To begin, sit in a chair, but you can try other postures as you wish, like sitting on a cushion on the floor, or lying down. It's a good idea to close your eyes as it will help you to concentrate better.

Always remember if any of the techniques, especially the breathing technique, make you feel in anyway dizzy then take smaller and shorter breaths.

If you wish, you can integrate meditation music playlists from YouTube or other sources into your meditation.

Sit in a comfortable chair in a quiet place where nothing will disturb you, for the full duration of this exercise. Rest your hands in your lap, and uncross your legs, placing your feet flat on the floor.

Now do nothing more than pay attention to your breath. Breathe in slowly through your nose and notice the cool temperature of the air.

Now slowly exhale through your nose, notice the temperature as you breathe out. How warm it is!

Continue to slowly breathe in and out through your nose 10 times and notice how the sensations change. Take nice slow deep breaths in and out, try not to think about anything other than your breath.

If your mind wanders, as it will, don't get frustrated just return to focusing on your breathing - in and out. Notice how focusing on your breathing affects your thoughts.

Note each thought or feeling as it passes by and immediately return to your breath.

Now shift your focus to your chest and feel how it rises and falls with each breath you take. Slowly breathe in to the count of five, and then slowly breathe out to the count of five. Do this ten times then return to your normal breathing.

Now shift your attention to your belly. Take a deep breath in, to the count of five, - watch how your chest and belly move - Take ten more breaths and watch how it changes the movement in your abdomen and your chest.

Then return to your normal breathing. Listen to the sounds in the room. Do they seem more intense? Notice how many different sounds you can hear, both inside and outside your body.

Once more return your awareness to your body. Does it feel more tense or relaxed? Does it feel more warm or cool?

Are there any parts of your body that seem tense or uncomfortable? Just notice the tension, and take another deep breath through your nose. Breathe through the location of tension or pain.

Now slowly breathe through your mouth. Notice how this changes the movement of your belly and your chest.

Repeat this deep breathing 10 times, counting the seconds as you breathe in and counting the seconds as you breathe out.

Shift your attention to your mouth and feel the cold air across your tongue as you breathe in. Now feel the warm air of your breath as you breathe out.

Shift your attention to the roof of your mouth and notice how different, the temperature feels.

Return to your natural pattern of breathing and notice any differences you feel. Are you more relaxed or more tense? Do you feel more tired or awake? Whatever you are feeling don't judge it. Just notice it and accept it and return to watching your breath.

Now bring this breathing exercise to a close.

Slowly look around the room, turning your head from one side to the other. Then slowly rise from your chair. Take a moment to see how you feel standing up and consciously breathe in and breathe out.

Slowly start to walk around and see if you can continue to be mindful of your breath as you return to your daily routines, whether it's working, walking, driving, washing the dishes, or waiting for someone.

That's the end of the first mindfulness breathing technique. It is an introduction to the rest of the meditations. You can do this exercise in just a few minutes or continue for as long as thirty minutes.

The longer you do it, the more peaceful and relaxed you will feel. This practices trains your mind to be still, but neurologically it's in a heightened state of awareness, the perfect situation from which to set about on any tasks that you need to do.

At any time in the future, if tension or anxiety show up in your life, use this breathing awareness technique to calm your mind and your body.

As you become more familiar with breathing awareness, feel free to vary it in anyway, like combining it with other meditation exercises or just watching how your mind responds as you consciously breathe in breathe out.

Meditation 2 Body Relaxing the Mind

The first meditation helps your mind to relax your body. This next technique will help your body to relax your mind.

This technique is often called progressive muscle relaxation or sometimes it is called total body relaxation. It is particularly effective for people who are unusually tense, and is excellent for reducing stress and anxiety. It is also useful in helping with pain relief in a variety of neurological and physical disorders.

You can use this technique at night if you want to go into a deep sleep.

Progressive muscle relaxation is very easy to do. Basically you just tighten and then relax each muscle group in your body, and in between you use the breathing technique. This exercise is best done on a warm mat, or you can do it in a very comfortable chair.

So let's go to the Progressive Muscle Relaxation exercise: - First take a deep breath, hold it as long as you can, then breathe out as much air as possible. Then hold your breath as long as you can before inhaling. Repeat this five times.

Next take a deep breath in, and as you do this, tense all the muscles in your body from head to toe, and hold them as long as you possibly can, (most people can do this for about 10 to 20 seconds). Then relax everything, expelling the air from your lungs. Do this three more times. Then breathe out and relax the muscles in your body.

Take another deep breath and starting at the top of your head tighten up all of your face then let it go as you breathe out.

Breathe in, deeply scrunch up your forehead and hold for five seconds, then release breathing out.

Breathe in, tighten your mouth and jaw, and hold for five seconds and release as you breathe out.

Now stretch your mouth open, as wide as you can. (If there is any sign of cramp, stop immediately). Hold your mouth open for five seconds and release. Take another deep breath and yawn, and release all of the tension in your face.

Take a deep breath in, pull your shoulders up toward your head, and tighten all of the muscles in your neck. Hold for five seconds then push your shoulders plus down as you exhale. Slowly roll your head from side to side as you fully and completely relax.

Take another deep breath in and tighten your arms and your hands. Clench your fist tightly and hold on tight as long as you can. Breathe out and relax your arms and hands, while splaying out your fingers.

Breathe in, push your arms into the chair or floor, and hold for 10 seconds and release, breathing out. Shake out your own hands and arms then take another deep breath, yawn take a few moments to sense the relaxation in your upper body and face.

Next take a breath and tighten your stomach muscles. Hold them for a count of 10 then relax, pushing all the air out of your lungs.

Push your stomach out, pull it in again, push it out again, and then let all of your tension go. Repeat the pushing and pulling 10 times.

Take another deep breath. Tighten your buttocks, hold them as long as you can then breathe out and relax.

Breathe in, tighten your upper legs, and then quickly relax as you breathe out.

Breathe in tighten your calves; hold for five seconds then release as you breathe out.

Breathe in again, scrunch up your toes, hold and release, then stretch them upward and apart as you slowly breathe out all the air in your lungs.

Now shake your feet and legs as fast as you can for another 10 seconds, then rest.

Yawn and spend a few moments feeling the relaxation flowing through your legs and body. Once more take a huge breath in, tighten your entire body, and hold for 10 seconds, then release as you force all the air out of your lungs.

Now do a full body scan. Feel how relaxed your face is... then your neck...your shoulders, your arms...your chest... your stomach...your back... your legs, and finally your feet. If any part feels tense, then breathe through it again.

Lie there for a few minutes and gently stretch.
When you feel ready, slowly stand up and slowly walk around, feeling how each part of your body moves. Take it easy for a few minutes ...you're very relaxed at this point.

You can do this meditation morning, noon or night and it is a wonderful way to relax, or to go for a power nap or into a deep sleep.

Meditation 3 Healing your Stressors

As I mentioned earlier, Mindfulness Meditation (MM) practice is about concentrating on your breath, being mindful for short periods of time every day, until eventually these periods get longer and you start to relax and enjoy the Present even more.

When you begin to meditate, you will notice that your mind starts to wander; thoughts keep coming up and floating by, interrupting your breathing concentration. Just let them be and every time you get lost in thoughts, just note them, and gently return to your breath.

To stay focused on the breath try making a soft mental note like "in" and "out", while you experience and concentrate fully on your breath. Or as you breathe in and out, count your breaths from one to ten and every time you get distracted by a thought, start again at one.

It will take a lot of practice before you reach ten while focused only on your breath, without getting distracted by thoughts.

Forgiving yourself for wandering and starting over again is a big part of the meditation. Beginning again and again is the practice; it's not a problem to overcome, so that one day you will do "real" meditation. You are continually building your meditation muscle.

Before we start this meditation, I want you to think of three situations or stressors that are distressing to you now or have been in the past. These could be related to people, to places, to events, to loss, to abandonment, to work, to relationships, to finances or any other situations that are problematic for you.

These stressors could be from your past, or something that is distressing you now at this present moment, or it might be something that you feel could be problematic in the future.

For now, just think of the three situations. We will bring these into the meditation as we go along.

You may have more than three stressors in your life. However, we will only focus on three for now. You can include the others over time, when you practice this at home, at any time of day, while looking at all parts of your life.

Remember, you can do these meditations anywhere, at any time; in your kitchen, in bed, in the garden or during a break at work.

Lying down is not a good idea, unless you really want to fall asleep, and then these meditations can be used as an aid to sleep.

To start, find a place where you will be comfortable for several minutes and where you will not be disturbed.

Settle in to your chair or mat, feeling relaxed, your back straight but not tense.

Turning first to your breath, notice your breathing, as you breathe in and as you breathe out.

Breathing in and breathing out.

Notice each breath as a unique experience, watching as the lungs fill, as you breathe in and noticing as they fall back, as you breathe out.

Breathing in, breathing out.

In this meditation I will ask you to notice the three situations that have been disturbing or distressing to you, either in the past or something that is distressing you currently. Even something that in the future might be problematic.

As we go through the meditation, I will ask you to notice these situations one at a time allowing you to feel any emotions that arise as part of these situations.

You are not going to avoid or reject these emotions, but you are going to become aware of them, integrate and accept them, as a way to better deal with them.

This will allow you to release them and let them go.

Breathing in, breathing out.

Notice as you breathe how your belly moves ever so slightly with each breath.

Now I want you to focus in your solar plexus area. Visualise or imagine a golden globe of warmth and energy residing there, which is healing and soothing, which is radiating energy throughout your body as you breathe in and as you breathe out.

Picture this golden globe emanating heat and healing to every fibre in your body, as you breathe in and breathe out.

Picture this globe as being with you all the time every day as you go about your daily chores.

Breathing in, breathing out.

Picture this globe as giving you healing energies which you can draw on at any time.

Picture yourself as healthy and strong.

Picture your body as functioning well.

Breathing in, breathing out.

And repeat to yourself "I am healthy and strong", "I am healthy and strong".

And now, calling up into your mind the first situation or stressor that you would like to deal with;
Picturing the situation, the people, picturing the thoughts, and allowing yourself to feel the feelings and emotions that arise, in response to this situation. Allow those emotions to well-up inside your body and inside your mind.

Know that these emotions are normal and human and cannot hurt or harm you as long as you accept them. Remember not to avoid or reject them. No matter what the feelings are, whether it is fear, shame, guilt, sadness or anger. Feel those feelings fully and completely.

Breathing in, breathing out.

Allow these emotions to percolate inside of you and as you do this they will eventually reduce. Allow these emotions to gradually fade and get smaller and allow yourself to let them go.

They will integrate into your energy field and lose their power. They will not be creating or perpetuating physical or psychological symptoms inside you, any more.

Turning now to your breathing; breathing in, breathing out. Notice your breath every time you breathe in and every time you breathe out.

Watch as the lungs fill with air and watch as they fall back.

Notice the abdomen as it moves in and out as you breathe.

And picture once again this golden globe of energy, healing and wellbeing, located in the middle of your body, your solar plexus, as it radiates warmth and healing energies to every fibre and cell of your body.

Repeat to yourself "I am healthy and strong", "I am healthy and strong".

And turn now to the second issue or stressful situation that you'd like to call up and deal with. Allow yourself to think about this and notice it and to feel any emotions connected to it, no matter what they are; no matter how deep they are, allowing them to well up inside of you.

Fear, sadness, anger, guilt and shame; they are all normal emotions that everyone feels.

Allow these emotions to well up inside you and to percolate throughout your body and your mind. They can't hurt you or harm you as long as you don't resist them or try to repress them.

Feel them fully and completely and know that as all emotions do, they will tend to fade and fall away.

Breathing in, breathing out.

And now allow these emotions to get smaller as you gradually let them go and release them. They will not be causing or perpetuating physical or psychological symptoms any longer.

Turn back again now to your breathing; breathing in and breathing out, breathing in and breathing out.

As you notice each breath, as the lungs fill with air, as you breathe in and as they fall back as you breathe out, as the belly moves in and out with each breath.

Notice once again the golden globe of warmth and wellness and health that you have, that you hold – as it radiates healing energy throughout your body. It will keep you healthy and well.

Breathing in, breathing out.

And repeat to yourself, "I am healthy and strong", "I am healthy and strong".

Turn now to the third situation or issue you would like to deal with today and thinking about it, noticing it and allowing any emotions or feelings that are associated with it to well up inside of you, and allowing them to come into your heart and your mind and your body.

Feel them fully and completely no matter what they are, no matter how deep they are; know that you can tolerate them. Do not trying to resist or reject them, allow them to percolate within your body, allowing yourself to feel them completely, without fear, because they cannot harm you or hurt you.

Breathing in, breathing out.

Know that these emotions, as all emotions do, will gradually fade away and fall away.
Allow these emotions now to ebb, to get smaller and to be released, letting them go as you turn your attention once again to your breath.

Breathing in, breathing out, breathing in and breathing out.

Notice your lungs again as the fill and expand and as they fall back.

Notice your belly as it moves, rises and falls with each in and out-breath.

Turn your attention once again to the golden globe, the ball of health and healing energy in your belly region that you have. It keeps you well and radiates healing energy. Picture it sending healing energy rays to every part of your body, to every cell and every fibre in your body as you breathe in and breathe out.

Picture your body right now as healthy and strong.

Picture yourself able to do anything that you'd like.

Picture yourself as well and healthy.
Repeat to yourself once again "I am healthy and strong", "I am healthy and strong".

Take this meditation with you throughout the day. Picture the golden globe of wellbeing, remembering to be kind to yourself and others, every day.

Remember to be forgiving of yourself every day, recognising that emotions will come and go, stressful situations will come and go, but that you can deal with them by recognising these emotions. Do not allow them to be held inside and causing physical or psychological pain.

Breathing in, breathing out.

Take a few deeper breaths right now and whenever you're ready, open your eyes, ready to meet whatever comes today.

Meditation 4 – Yawning

Yawning is a very effective way of relaxing your mind and body. A good yawn increases your awareness, alertness, and bodily relaxation. It will relax you in minutes.

Find a quiet, comfortable place where you can stand and won't be disturbed by others. Stand in a place where your arms are free to swing side to side. You can sit, but standing allows you to achieve a fuller inhalation.

Begin by taking a very deep breath and stretching your mouth wide open. Think as if you were in the dentist and have to open your mouth as wide as possible. If you feel a cramp coming on, stop immediately.

As you exhale, make a long, sighing aaaagh sound. Don't worry if you don't feel like yawning or don't believe you can. Keep trying and by the fifth or sixth fake yawn you'll eventually feel a real one coming on.

Pay close attention to what happens in your mouth, your throat, your chest and belly, and don't be surprised if your eyes start watering or you see 'stars'.

Allow yourself about ten to twelve yawns and pause for a few seconds between each one. The total time for this exercise should be about two minutes.

Yawning is contagious. Ever notice when you hear and see someone else yawn, it will stimulates the same response in you?

Conscious yawning generates a deep sense of relaxation, calmness, and alertness, and like the previous meditation, it stimulates a unique circuit in the brain that enhances consciousness, the key to any contemplative or spiritual practice.

Yawn before you tackle a difficult problem, and yawn when you find yourself in a conflict with another person. Yawning will help reduce stress, literally in a matter of minutes.

It is preferable to do it in the privacy of your home; otherwise people might mistakenly think you are bored or tired.

Meditation 5 – Focus on a Mantra

A mantra is a repeated word, phrase, or prayer that makes you feel happy, peaceful, and calm. Repeat it as you breathe slowly and deeply.

You can also recite brief prayers, passages from a spiritual text or sayings that are special to you. It has to be personally meaningful to you – it doesn't matter where it originated, whether it's religious or non religious.

Mere repetition of any phrase will reduce stress, anxiety and anger, while improving one's quality of life.

To begin, find a comfortable place where you won't be disturbed and close your eyes.

Take several deep breaths. As you exhale, silently, or with a whisper, say a word, phrase, or sound that gives you a feeling of serenity or joy – some words you can use; peace, love, patience, slow down, OM, God etc).

Stay with your breathing and the repetition of your personal mantra. Repeat the mantra slowly as you breathe in and out, for about ten to twenty minutes.

Acknowledge unwanted thoughts and let them go, returning to the repetition of your mantra.

Don't try to achieve any goal or state, just focus on your word for the full ten to twenty minutes. When you finish, sit quietly for a few minutes and then open your eyes. Yawn three or four times and slowly move about the room.

Try this for a few weeks. You will notice how much calmer, less anxious and more receptive you are. Change your mantra as often as you like, paying attention to how different ones affect your awareness and behaviour.

Meditation 6 – Visualization and Guided Imagery

The more you visualise a spiritual or emotional state, or a specific goal in life, the easier it is for your brain to materialize that intention into your inner and outer reality.

To experience the benefits of visualisation, choose any place, imaginary or real, that feels beautiful and relaxing; for example, a beach, a mountaintop, a waterfall, or a sailboat on a lake.

Visualise the tiny details on the ground and in the sky? If you're at work and feeling especially pressured and tense, you can take a three-minute "vacation" to calm any mental disturbance in your frontal lobes by simply recalling a pleasant memory.

If you wish, you can visualise a loved one, or a romantic scene. Let your fantasies take you to wherever they want to go. And, if you find that you have trouble visualising, yawn a few times, because it stimulates an important part of the visualization process in your brain.

Imagination is what the brain does best, and pleasurable fantasies are its best source of food.

See how well you can visualise the following scenario, commonly used in stress-relaxation programs.

Find a quiet place to lie or sit down. Close your eyes and take five deep breaths, followed by four or five yawns.

Take another deep breath and visualise yourself lying on a warm, sunny beach.

Feel the sun radiating through your skin and warming the muscles underneath.

Feel yourself sinking into the warm soft sand as you become more and more relaxed. Take another deep breath and feel yourself melting into the beach. Stay with this image for two or three minutes, and let your imagination take you wherever it wants to go.

Now, imagine yourself walking through a thick, humid, tropical forest. Take a deep breath and feel the warm damp air blow across your face.

Visualise the path, surrounded by lush, green, tropical plants. Listen to the birds chirping in the trees. What do they sound like? What do they look like? What colours do you see?

As you walk down the path, you come around a bend. There, in front of you, is the most beautiful waterfall in the world. Watch how the water spills down the side of the mountain, over the rocks, and into a crystal clear pool of water. Watch a salmon leap in the air.

Now step into the pool. Take a deep breath and feel the warm tropical water washing over your feet as you slowly step into the waterfall pool.

As you step further in and under the waterfall, feel the clear, warm water gently flow down over your head, washing away all of your tension and cares. Take three deep breaths, and with each exhalation, let the water wash all of your worries away.

Now, feel our body melting into the pool. As you breathe in deeply, feel yourself turning into a stream. As you and the water become one, you begin to slowly flow down the stream.

Feel the sun shining overhead as you float down the river, far, far away from all of the tensions of the world. Watch where the river takes you, and continue the inner journey as far as it wants to go. When your journey is finished, notice how relaxed you feel.

When creating your personalised "vacation," or when guiding a friend through these visualisations, remember to use repetitive words and phrases that evoke relaxation; words like: warm, soft, deep, heavy, etc.

For example, tell yourself that you are "feeling more and more relaxed..... Going deeper and deeper into relaxation....arms feeling warm and heavy and relaxed....." The repetition lulls you into a trancelike state of peace.

Visualisation is an important aspect for setting any goal, since much of your unconscious brain is oriented around a visual construction of the world. As we know from many Olympic athletes, visualising their performance actually improves their game.

The same is true for work. If you visualise a possible solution to a problem, the problem is more easily solved because it specifically activates cognitive circuits involved with working memory.

Visualisation can also help us distance ourselves from a disturbing memory or problem, yet it simultaneously brings us closer to our desires.

If you visualize a sacred or spiritual symbol, it reinforces your religious beliefs. You can visualise yourself being a better golfer, or you can envision yourself as being a more ethical person, but in either case, your neural connections will help you actually achieve those goals.

Meditation 7 – Candle Meditation

With this meditation, begin by placing a candle on table, and sit on a comfortable chair with your feet flat on the floor. Smells can enhance meditation experiences, so a scented candle may be used. Have a lighter or matches in your hand.

Take a few deep breaths and yawn, just focusing on the unlit candle. Then, in slow motion, light the candle, and take another deep breath. Slowly put the lighter down, and sitting up straight, begin to gaze at the candle. Blink as little as possible.

Bring your focus to the flame. Let it fill your entire consciousness as you observe how it dances and flutters. What colours does it make? Does the flame grow taller, and then get smaller? Keep watching all of the qualities of the flame for three or four minutes, while breathing in and out consciously.

If interruptive thoughts come into your mind, acknowledge them and let them go, and bring your focus back to the candle flame.

Now close your eyes and visualise the flame in your mind. Watch how it dances and flutters in your imagination.

If the image of the flame fades, open your eyes, study the flame, and then close your eyes again. Keep doing this until you hold the image of the flame in your mind for five minutes with your eyes closed.

It's simple, powerful, and enjoyable. Each time you do this meditation, try to extend the time. You can also use your imagination to become one with the candle. To do this, you imagine the flame coming closer and closer to your closed eyes. Then you imagine that you're inside the flame.

In another variation, imagine the flame burning away all of your thoughts, desires, and problems: anger, stress, impatience, greed, etc.

You can also use other objects – a pretty rock or a crystal, or an interesting leaf, to immerse your attention upon.

Breathing meditation teaches you to become aware of your inner state and body, whereas object meditations, like this candle exercise, train your mind to become more observant of the outside world.

Meditation 8 - Walking Meditation

Walking is a well-established technique for enhancing physical fitness. You can also make it a part of your daily brain-enhancement program. All you need to do is to bring attention to the act of taking a single step.

The following is a traditional Buddhist walking meditation, a mindfulness meditation. The exercise requires concentrated attention and awareness, so watch out for that inner critic who is always in a rush.

If you experience any balance or co-ordination problems, do not try this exercise without assistance from a friend.

First, find a place, without obstacles, where you can walk for about ten or twenty paces. A long hallway will do, or a lawn or open park, but try to find a quiet and pleasant spot, like a garden.

Stand up and gently shift your weight back and forth between each foot. But take your time. Notice at what point the heel of one foot comes off the ground, and notice how your weight shifts onto the various parts of your other foot.

Do you have more weight on the balls of your feet, on the side, or on your heel? Continue to shift your weight back and forth for at least sixty seconds.

Now with your two feet on the ground, slowly shift your weight forward and backward, and notice what happens in your toes. What does your big toe do as you move? Your little toe? Repeat this for another minute.

Continue to shift your weight forward and backward, but turn your attention to the part of your body that makes you shift. Is it in your ankles? Your calves? Your hips? Notice how hard it is to identify where the movement comes from, and continue to rock for another minute.

Next, in slow motion, begin to take a single step forward. But only lift your heel a couple of inches. In which muscle does the step begin? In your foot or leg or knee? Raise your heel ten times.

Now change to the other foot and lift your heel another ten times. Notice how different it feels. Shift your attention to your knee, and notice how it feels.

Slowly, very slowly, lift your foot a few inches from the ground, and pay attention to the subtle body adjustments that must be made for balance.

Lower your foot to the ground and raise the other foot two inches. Continue to alternate twenty times as you study which parts of your body are involved. What happens in your hips? How much does your body sway? How does it make you feel to move so slowly and deliberately? Notice any judgements, take a deep breath, and let them go.

Now begin to take slow steps forward, four steps with every breath in, four steps with every breath out. After a few minutes, take three steps with each inhalation and exhalation.

Do this for another two minutes, and then try taking only two steps as you slowly breathe in, and two more steps as you exhale. Do this in reverse if you find it easier.

Practice integrating your breathing with your walking for the next five minutes, walking as slowly as you can.

When you reach the end of the hall or yard (or after about twenty steps), turn around in slow motion. Take two minutes to turn around, watching how your balance works, and then slowly walk back to where you began.

At first, each step will feel uncoordinated, but as you become aware of how your feet, legs, hips, back, and shoulders move, your steps will become more fluid.

The longer you practice, the more you'll become aware of the texture of the ground, the colours of the grass, the sound of people talking, and the exquisite movements of your body. Whatever you perceive, focus on it, and then come back to your breathing and take another step.

To fully appreciate the power of walking meditation, do it with a partner or friend. With just a little practice, you'll find that you can take your relaxation with you anywhere.

From a spiritual perspective, walking meditation also encourages you to bring your inner values into play with the world, thus helping you experience daily life with greater depth and unity. It will also help you to develop patience.

Meditation 9 – Memory Enhancement

This mediation includes making four different sounds that can be sung, or said, and while you make the sounds, you touch different fingers for each sound.

The addition of movement and singing to any meditation significantly enhances the brain's performance.

Sing or say the sounds sa, ta, na, and ma as you touch your thumb on both hands with each of your fingers in turn. Take a moment and try it now.

Using both hands, touch your thumb and index finger when you say SA, your thumb and middle finger when you say ta, your thumb and ring finger when you say na, and your thumb and small finger when you say ma. Now you are ready to begin.

Start by finding a comfortable place where you can sit upright with good posture. Take two minutes to focus on your breathing, watching how your chest rises and falls.

Begin saying the sounds sa, ta, na, ma out loud while you touch your fingers in succession on both hands. Continue for two minutes.

Next, repeat the sounds in a whisper while continuing the finger movements. You can still say it, but just in a whisper. Do this for another two minutes.

Now, repeat the sounds internally. Say them silently to yourself while continuing the finger movements and do this for four minutes.

Repeat the sounds in a whisper for another two minutes as you continue to touch your fingers on both hands.

Finally, say the sounds out loud for the final two minutes as you touch your fingers in succession. Then rest and pay attention to how you feel.

It has been proven scientifically, that continuous practice of this meditation can create a huge improvement in memory function.

Instead of sa, ta, na and ma, you can create variations on this meditation. Choose four different words – peace, happiness, compassion, and joy – and touch each finger as you say the words out loud while walking.

Then take each word and spell them out on your fingers. With peace, after you touch your four fingers for the first four letters, touch the first finger again for the letter e.

Then spell it again, starting with the second finger. If you try it, you'll see that it requires intense concentration, but that too is the key to making neurological changes in the brain.

You can modify any meditation to suit your interest or needs, and it will still enhance the overall function of your brain.

Meditation 10 - Forgiveness Meditation

This powerful meditation is about sending kindness and forgiveness to others. It is very powerful and may transform your physical and emotional life.

It doesn't take much effort to practice this forgiveness meditation, and if you make a commitment to do it a few minutes every day, you'll rewire your brain for your mental and physical benefit. It will help to prevent current and future pain in your life and to reduce any reoccurrence of addiction.

The characteristic of an unforgiving heart usually begins with resentment and holding a grudge. You become inwardly bitter and pre-occupied with hate and self pity. You just can't come to terms with what was done to you or in some cases, said about you.

You want revenge, you want to punish the offender but the only one being punished is you, by you. You will continue to live with the painful side effects of these strong emotions until you make a decision to forgive. Forgiveness is a cure and also the future prevention of these side effects.

Repression or suppression of what we feel is almost always unconscious, especially when we are young because the emotional pain seems too great to take on board. We push it down and start to fill our reservoir of repressed emotions, but they come out in many other ways; irritability, anxiety, chronic pain and addiction, as mentioned earlier.

Most people, who have suffered abuse as a child, whether it is physical, emotional or sexual abuse, repress it. They cannot believe that a parent, a trusted friend or relative would do such a thing, so they live in denial, often blaming themselves.

Total forgiveness is not achieved by repressing what has happened. You can only reach total forgiveness when you reveal and heal the reality, when you come to terms with what happened; that this person actually did or said this, and then we have to forgive them, for our sakes.

Forgiving does not mean to be blind to what happened. Forgiveness means you have to see and feel what happened and then set the perpetrator free or you will never be at peace.

The wrong, the evil done to you is then acknowledged, we are not blind to it, and we are not pretending it didn't happen.

The only way back to sanity and peace of mind is to reveal and remember everything in a safe environment with a trusted friend or maybe a counsellor and then use the forgiveness meditation.

Telling someone with the purpose of hurting another's credibility or reputation is just another form of seeking revenge. Avoid this at all costs and only share to heal your pain and not to hurt another, no matter what they have done.

Share with another for your health's sake and not to make the offender look bad or to punish them in the eyes of another.

Most of the people we must forgive do not believe they have done anything wrong and often believe whatever they did, was justifiable.

Forgiveness is for your benefit and remember that reconciliation with the other person may never happen, but you will have moved on with your life.

Deep hurts may never be fully eradicated. The truth is they did happen. We cannot easily forget that, but we must reveal and heal them and no longer dwell on them, stopping them creating physical and emotional problems in our life.

You need to face up to the seriousness of what happened and still forgive, for your sake.

You have to be aware of the evil that you chose to forgive. You have to stop covering up what someone has done to you, excusing them and refusing to see what was wrong. This is living in denial.

You have to come to terms with the reality of what happened. We do not need to pretend that we are not hurt when we have been betrayed, molested, unjustly criticized or injured in other ways.

We need to share these hurts with another and then forgive the perpetrator so that we never allow them to control our lives and our relationships with others.

Keep doing the forgiveness meditation until the perpetrator has no power to cause you pain any more.

Total forgiveness is difficult and may be painful for a while. It often hurts when we kiss revenge goodbye. It hurts to think that the other person may be getting away with what they did and nobody knowing about it. But when you acknowledge fully what they did, share it and forgive, your life will move into a different realm and will take on a new meaning.

Forgiveness is a choice, a painful choice at first, an act of will, not of feeling. You must do it, not just think about it, and when you do it, you stop any resentment growing.

The desire for punishment and revenge disturbs us, keeps us bound to the perpetrator and keeps us wrapped in anger. Only when this desire subsides through forgiveness will we have peace of mind and peace of body.

Maybe for the first time, your focus will be on your life and how to make it better, and not on the perpetrators and what they did to you. It will set you free to live your life.

When you forgive, you rid yourself of bitterness and give up the desire to get revenge and to punish.

Bitterness is an excessive desire for revenge that comes from deep resentment and keeps you angry, irritable, causing high blood pressure, sleeplessness, depression, negativity and generally feeling unwell.

Bitterness also drives people away from you as no one can get close to a negative person.

Forgiveness is good for your physical and emotional wellbeing and for your healthy relationship with others, so forgive yourself, forgive God and forgive others.

Forgiveness helps you to preserve your dignity and restore your self-esteem. It is a life-long commitment.

In the meditation that follows, you will wish the perpetrator well, applying the Golden Rule; what you want for yourself you also want for them, that you want them forgiven just as you would want forgiveness if the roles were reversed.

Your suffering may never abate until you go through this process.

For many people the prayer known to many Christians as the "Our Father" sums it up well, where it says forgive us only as we forgive others.

For people who have been abused, 'Forgive us" could be replaced with "Heal us". It will be very challenging to do this. Mahatma Gandhi said "The weak can never forgive. Forgiveness is the attribute of the strong".

The greater the hurt perpetrated against you, the greater the transformation in your life when you forgive. Look upon forgiveness as an opportunity to heal your life. Consider it a challenge and grasp it with both hands.

Whether what was done to you was deliberate or not, you were hurt. Many children when they grow up will realize that their parents have failed them in some area and they will need to forgive them. We must forgive everyone we feel anger towards because it is we, not they, who are in need.

Forgiving an enemy or someone who has abused you is the highest level of spirituality that exists and it has produced miraculous results in many people's lives.

You need to become willing first and then to have sufficient motivation, one of which might be the emotional and physical devastation that 'not forgiving' is causing you.

When someone has upset you, rather than repress your hurt and anger, causing you physical pain, try the forgiveness meditation. Remember that the structure of your brain can be damaged by anger, anxiety, and stress.

You might be surprised at the amount of resistance you may feel the first time you do this meditation. In fact, it may be the most difficult – yet most important – meditation for you in the world. It is part of most mindfulness training programs. It is also the cornerstone of every major religious tradition, the golden rule of loving your neighbour as you would love yourself.

Do not dismiss the importance that forgiveness plays when it comes to getting along with others and healing emotional and physical pain.

Forgiveness improves family relationships, decreases pain and depressive symptoms and it can heal a wounded romantic heart.

Even the act of choosing to replace an unforgiving attitude with a forgiving one affects the peripheral and central nervous systems in ways that promote physical and psychological health.

Take a moment to think about a person that has upset you, maybe someone that you feel a lot of anger towards. Imagine sending him or her love. It's not easy, is it?

Research has shown that victims of violent crime and war who can forgive their perpetrators have decreased pain, anxiety and depression, while those who can't forgive are more inclined toward physical and psychiatric disease.

The forgiveness meditation that follows involves picturing a series of people and sending them good vibes. While doing this, generate as clear a mental image of them as possible.

Begin by sitting quietly in a place where you will not be disturbed.

Starting with yourself, send love to yourself by repeating the following, a few times, silently to yourself:

"May I be happy, May I be well, May I be filled with kindness and peace".

Notice how this makes you feel!

If you feel unworthy or uncomfortable saying this to yourself, send love to someone you like – a friend or even a pet "May you be happy, may you be well, may you be filled with kindness and peace."

Keep repeating it until you are filled with a warm, compassionate attitude toward that person.

Now turn that energy around and direct it again to yourself: "May I be happy, may I be well, may I be filled with kindness and peace."
The necessity of generating self-love cannot be overstated.

Next, turn your attention to the person you love the most. Smile as you visualise his or her face and repeat "May you be happy, may you be well, may you be filled with kindness and peace."

Then return the love to yourself. "May I be happy, May I be well, May I be filled with kindness and peace"

Now move on to another person, perhaps a family member, or friend, and send that person your loving energy. "May you be happy, may you be well, may you be filled with kindness and peace."

See their faces in your mind's eye. Notice how your feelings change when you think about this person.

Keep enlarging your circle by generating love to as many different people as you can: work colleagues, neighbours, etc.

Keep saying silently to them "May you be happy, may you be well, may you be filled with kindness and peace."

Again notice how the feelings of sending love to others, changes your mood, how this makes you feel better.

Now extend your feelings to the people you find more difficult to love or forgive, people you are angry with. Say to each of them "May you be happy, May you be well, May you be filled with kindness and peace", sending a loving thought to those who are upsetting you or who have hurt you in the past.

This will be very hard to do this at first. Just acknowledge your feelings of reluctance and come back to loving yourself. In time it gets easier and easier to send love to those you don't like, or who make you angry. And you will start to feel better, and you will start loving yourself more, by forgiving others.

Remember the old saying "My condemnation injures me, my forgiveness sets me free".

If anyone seems very difficult to forgive, look for one small quality that you liked about them – perhaps his/her smile, or some other quality – and focus your entire attention on that single trait as you say "May you be happy, may you be well, may you be filled with kindness and peace."

Try to recall one kind thing he or she once did, and concentrate on that. Hold the positive thought as long as you can, saying "May you be happy, may you be well, may you be filled with kindness and peace", then notice if your feelings have changed. Do you feel less anger? Less hurt? Even the slightest decrease is beneficial to your brain and to healing your physical and emotional pain.

Then coming back to yourself say "May you be happy, may you be well, may you be filled with kindness and peace" as if someone else was saying it to you.

Then finish your meditation by extending your love, kindness, and forgiveness to the Universe. "May everyone be happy, may everyone be well, and may everyone be filled with kindness and peace ", while holding a vision in your mind of all the different people in the world, all cultures, all colours, all religions, and all political groups.
Imagine everyone getting along with each other and living together in peace.

This forgiveness meditation is very powerful and could completely change your life. During the day, when any person you dislike or who makes you angry, pops into your mind's eye, just send them good wishes with this healing phrase "May you be happy, may you be well, may you be filled with kindness and peace", and you will no longer be carrying them around in your head.

Keep saying it until the people who hurt or distressed you, have faded away and no longer have power to cause you pain or to control your life and your relationships.

So the next time someone upsets you, instead of killing off some neurons in your own brain, just send them this blessing "May you be happy, May you be well, May you be filled with kindness and peace". They probably need it more than you.

Forgiveness meditation improves the health of your brain and heart.
So if you now believe it is right for you to forgive and to move on with living your life, start this meditation.

Share your hurt with another person in a safe and confidential environment to reveal and heal your pain and never to hurt or damage another person's reputation.

Remember the Golden Rule, 'Do unto others as you would have them do unto you', if the roles were reversed. Be nice to people and start to live your own life, without the control or influence of past hurts.

Forgive yourself for your own human failings. If we don't forgive ourselves we lapse back into the trap of remembering the wrongs done by others and we will let fear and bitterness start to control our lives again.

Forgiving is a conscious act. Don't wait until it feels right or you may never do it. Act now. Do it because it is right, because it is good for you.

As Nelson Mandela said "Bitterness only hurts oneself. If you hate, you will give them your heart and your mind. Don't give those two things away."

Don't let anger and bitterness eat into your soul any longer.

Start this meditation and do it every time a memory of hurt comes into your mind. More memories will surface over time and you can now deal with them.

Those imaginary conversations of revenge and getting-even will subside, and your peace of mind will be restored. It will be very difficult to do at the start, but it gets easier and you will quickly see the benefits.

With forgiveness of ourselves and of others we let go of the past and its effect on our present. We restore our lives and move on from the wasted years of anger towards others that ruined our physical and emotional health. We start to accept ourselves as we are. We show mercy to the perpetrators of our hurt and free them from our lives.

CHAPTER 15 Final Reflections on Meditation

With meditation, only do what feels right for you. Otherwise, it becomes work. If it becomes a chore, you'll resist and resent it. After all, guilt will also hurt your brain. And the same applies to meditation. So the amount you practice is really up to you. The more you meditate, the greater the variety, the better.

Remember that exercise, social interaction, and optimism all tie for first place in terms of keeping your brain healthy. Meditation comes in second.

Meditate daily, and become expert in one of these mindfulness techniques.

When a sense of the absolute unity of all things happens, you might become aware that "you" are not your thoughts, and this raises the question of what "you" may actually be.

This can happen in any of the meditations we described before, but it typically results once you fully accept that the 'I' of you is the creator of everything in your life.

Be grateful for what you have. Gratitude for what you already have links your creative thoughts with the formless energy that permeates all life allowing you to create what you want.

Become a little more aware of life. Slow down by paying attention to your body movements and your breathing as you go about your daily activities.

Become more aware of how your mind produces an endless stream of unconscious feelings and thoughts. Become more aware of what you think, feel, say, and do.

Train your brain to become more organised and calm. With meditation, stress will diminish and life will begin to feel more pleasant and rich.

It's easy to be mindful throughout the day, and all you need to do is remind yourself to be aware.

You can take a minute to "meditate" in the elevator, when you're standing in line at the supermarket, when you're stuck in rush-hour traffic, or when you're gazing into the eyes of those you deeply love. This is what mindfulness is all about, and it will change your brain in beneficial ways.

CHAPTER 16 In Summary

A few years after I stopped drinking many of the unconscious repressed feelings going back to my childhood tried to reach the light of day, or come into my consciousness.

Because of my fear of their effect on my new life I tried to keep them repressed, however they created real physical pain in many parts of my body until I became aware of what was happening.

When I acknowledged and accepted that these feelings were the cause of the chronic pain, I cured the physical and emotional pain by talking to my brain and telling it what I knew.

Conscious recognition defeated the mind's diversion mechanism, which was triggered by the strong emotions in the unconscious reservoir trying to escape into consciousness.

The mind's earlier diversion of using alcoholism has also been cured in the same way, through awareness, knowledge and acceptance of the MindBody integration disorder that needed this diversion mechanism.

Following over 30 years of continuous sobriety in AA, because of my new awareness, knowledge and acceptance, I returned to social drinking successfully, without any addictive issues.

In those 30 years without alcohol I won many innovation awards and was featured on national TV. I received granted patents for some of my inventions. For ten of those years I ran my own company and designed a series of award-winning interactive animated products for teaching children how to learn through the medium of music.

Without alcohol I learned to achieve many dreams, including playing music, learning to dance, becoming an artist and inventor, and having fun.

I spent most of my life longing for joy, for approval only realising very late in life that it has to come first from the inside out.

Because of my many traumatic experiences I've been able to help many people who might otherwise have taken their own lives.

I'm a very optimistic person. I have had many trials and tribulations but deep down I feel very lucky to have figured out what was going on in my life, in my mind and in my body.

As a person believing I was unable to take a drink, I was not an easy person to live with, after I stopped taking alcohol. All of the repressed trauma, anger, fear, loss, grief and post-traumatic stress, combined with alcohol withdrawal made my life and the lives of those closest to me, challenging for many years.

I appreciate the period that I was off alcohol. It allowed me to find my true way. My realization of the cure for addiction means that that I can now enjoy alcohol without any addictive consequences.

I appreciated the joy in my life even more now that I know where the light comes from and how to keep it on.

I hope you enjoyed my book and that it benefits you or someone you know. The book is about emotions, about illness and about wellness; how they are related, and what you can do to enhance good health and combat physical and emotional pain in your life.

You will have gained a better understanding of how the brain can be responsible for the creation of very real physical and emotional pain and how you can do battle with your brain and stop the pain.

My story is backed by 40 years of medical research by the top Medical practitioners and Neuroscientists in the world today. I have no pain today. I have no addiction today.

I hope this book will help you to heal your life, no matter what challenges you face.

CHAPTER 17 The Program of Recovery

Remember, if your experience of life has included abuse, addiction, chronic pain, depression or attempted suicide, you don't need to hurt yourself any longer. You might want to, but you will never need to.

One day at a Time, make contact with an OTI member and go to a meeting. If no meeting is available then set one up.

When you come back from addiction, chronic pain, or the brink of suicide, you may need someone to hold your hand and walk you back into life.

If you feel there never was a point in your life when you felt okay, then the OTI program will bring you forward on a journey of recovery.

OTI is not allied with any sect or religious organization and it is totally up to you if you want to have a spiritual power in your life.

The emotions that we share at OTI meetings, under past or current traumatic or stressful events, will include: hurt, shame, anxiety, resentment, embarrassment, pain, anger, guilt, humiliation, fear, worry or other negative emotions. These will include everything going back as far as your childhood, including physical, sexual or emotional abuse.

Letters can be written to the abusers and read out at meetings and then destroyed. At the end of a meeting each member shares their gratitude list.

The OTI meeting is a safe space where you can express your feelings and then let them go. These emotions can be shared at the meeting and also written down between meetings for additional sharing.

The OTI Program works. When you attend an online or local meeting, with like-minded people who have reached the same level of despair and recovered, the results can be very powerful and life-affirming.

Going to an OTI meeting is not mandatory but it will make your life journey more pleasant, being able to converse and identify with people like yourself. It will help you to build a new, fulfilling and happy life and to share your journey with others.

OTI Meeting Format

A meeting can be held anywhere; in a private room or in member's homes, as long as the venue location is confidential and safe. An online OTI group is also being developed. The meeting should be self-sustaining through voluntary contributions.

Open the meeting with one of the Mindfulness Meditations (MM) from the previous chapter.

Then read The Preamble.

The Preamble:
OTI is an open, anonymous, confidential meeting where men and women heal through sharing their life stressors, their emotional and physical pain, with hope and belief for a new non addicted and pain free journey through life. OTI is not connected to any sect, denomination, politics, religion, organization or institution. Our primary purpose is to help each other to reveal and heal the issues that cause us emotional and physical pain, and to start on a new life journey together, one day at a time, achieving a fulfilling and happy life.

Before the Meeting Starts, announce:
"Whatever you share here, let it stay here". Everyone who wishes to, can share. Those who don't wish to share can say "I will pass today".

People who are deemed to speak for too long will be interrupted by the Chair of the meeting. A timer can be used if the group agrees to it.

All decisions must be made by the Group. Individuals do not have any power or control in OTI and service positions of Secretary and Chairperson must rotate every three months.

The Steps of OTI

1. Accepted that we are over the influence of addiction and chronic pain in all its manifestations, that we are now in control of our own lives.
2. Made a decision not to harm or injure ourselves or others, one day at a time
3. Made a searching and fearless inventory of our past lives and accepted that everything in our lives today is exactly as it was meant to be, that nothing happens in this world by mistake.
4. Admitted to another human being the exact details of our life, past and present.
5. Learned to relax through practising Mindfulness Meditation (MM) every day.
6. Made amends to those we had harmed and became honest in all our dealings
7. Apologized immediately when we were wrong and learned to be patient with others.
8. Continued to expand our joy helping others and ourselves, to our new abundant life
9. Went to OTI meetings (local or online) and shared our life story openly with other OTI members.
10. Refrained from taking mind-altering drugs
11. Stopped searching in the past by switching on the light of this new MindBody awareness.
12. Forgave ourselves and others, and became willing to live in the Present.

Powerlessness and Unmanageability are no longer a part of your new pain free and non-addicted life.

If you would like set up and register your OTI
Meeting please send an email to jchesnan@gmail.com.

Some Prayers for the spiritually inclined

This book is not allied with any sect, spiritual or religious organization. However If you have a spiritual or religious leaning, then start each day by reading the 'Just for Today' prayer and then hand your will and your life into the care and direction of your God with the 'Handing Over', prayer. You can add in the other prayers; 'Prayer of St Francis' and 'Clearing Prayer' as you wish.

Just For Today

Just for today I will make no attempt to harm or kill myself. I will always call someone if this thought arises.

Just for today I will contact another OTI member, either online or in person and share my thoughts, my fears and my hopes.

Just for today I will be willing to give time and listen to another OTI member

Just for today I will find out about OTI meetings, online and face to face and commit to attending at least one per week.

I will live through this day only, and not try to tackle all my problems at once. I can do something for twelve hours that would appal me if I felt I had to keep it up for a lifetime.

Just for today I will be happy. I accept that most people are as happy as they make up their minds to be.

Just for today I will adjust myself to what is, and not try to adjust everything to my own desires. I will take my luck as it comes, and fit myself to it.

Just for today I will try to strengthen my mind. I will study. I will learn something useful. I will not be a mental loafer. I will read something that requires effort, thought and concentration.

Just for today I will exercise my soul in three ways: I will do somebody a good turn and not get found out; if anyone knows of it, it will not count. I will do at least two things I don't want to do – just for exercise. I will not show anyone that my feelings are hurt; they may be hurt, but today I will not show it.

Just for today I will get up at a reasonable time and hand my will and my life into the care of God or a higher power of my own understanding. I will accept that whatever happens today is for my good.

Just for today I will be agreeable. I will look as well as I can, dress well, keep my voice low, be courteous, criticize not one bit. I won't find fault with anything or anyone, nor try to improve or regulate anybody but myself.

Just for today I will have a plan. I may not follow it exactly, but I will have it. It will save me from two pests: hurry and indecision.

Just for today I will have a quiet half hour all by myself and relax. During this half hour, I will try to get a better perspective of my life.

Just for today I will be unafraid. Especially I will not be afraid to notice what is beautiful and to believe that as I give to the world, so the world will give to me.

Just for today I will count my blessings. I will list all the things in my life that I am grateful for.

Just for today I will practice forgiveness of myself and others.

At the end of each day I will thank God, or a higher power of my own understanding, for getting me through this day.

Prayer of St Francis

Lord, make me an instrument of Thy Peace. Where there is hatred, let me sow love; where there is injury, let me sow pardon; where there is doubt, let me sow faith; where is despair, let me sow hope; where there is darkness, let me sow light; and where there is sadness, let me sow joy. O, Divine Master, grant that I may not so much seek to be consoled, as to console; to be understood, as to understand; to be loved, as to love; for it is in giving that we receive; it is in pardoning that we are pardoned, and it is in dying that we are born to eternal life.

Handing Over Prayer

God, I hand my will and my life into your care and direction today. I offer myself to you to do with me as thou wilt. Relieve me of the bondage of my false self that I may better do Thy will and return to my true self, which is happy, loving, joyful and free. Take away my difficulties, so that victory over them may bear witness to those I would help, of Thy power, Thy Love, and Thy Way of life. Relieve me of the bondage of self and the repetition of any hereditary ills. May I do Thy will always.

Clearing Prayer

God, I am now willing that you should have all of me, good and bad. I pray that you now remove from me every single defect of character which stands in the way of my usefulness to you, to me and to my fellows. Grant me strength, as I go out from here, to do your bidding. May my thoughts and the expression of my thoughts (words) be always pure and positive so that the materials with which they build be always good and for my benefit and create joy and abundance in all areas of my life. I accept that I have to change if I want the results in my life to change.

ABOUT THE AUTHOR

John Hesnan is an award winning patents granted Inventor and Entrepreneur. John's passions are; art, healing, writing, inventing, education and music.

www.ingramcontent.com/pod-product-compliance
Lightning Source LLC
Chambersburg PA
CBHW060257290526
45789CB00001B/340